How to Treat People

How to Treat People

A Nurse at Work

MOLLY CASE

VIKING
an imprint of
PENGUIN BOOKS

VIKING

UK | USA | Canada | Ireland | Australia
India | New Zealand | South Africa

Viking is part of the Penguin Random House group of companies
whose addresses can be found at global.penguinrandomhouse.com.

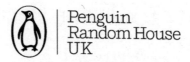

First published 2019
001

The publisher is grateful to quote from the following:
p. 89, 'Tulips' from *Collected Poems* by Sylvia Plath © 1960, 1965, 1971, 1981
by the Estate of Sylvia Plath. Reproduced here by permission of Faber and Faber Ltd.

p. 274, 'To My Daughter' by Stephen Spender. Reproduced with permission
of Curtis Brown Group Ltd, London, on behalf of the Estate of Stephen Spender.
Copyright © The Estate of Stephen Spender 1953.

Set in 12.5/14.75 pt Dante MT Std
Typeset by Jouve (UK), Milton Keynes
Printed and bound in Great Britain by Clays Ltd, Elcograf S.p.A.

A CIP catalogue record for this book is available from the British Library

ISBN: 978–0–241–34737–9

www.greenpenguin.co.uk

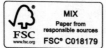

MIX
Paper from
responsible sources
FSC
www.fsc.org   FSC® C018179

Penguin Random House is committed to a
sustainable future for our business, our readers
and our planet. This book is made from Forest
Stewardship Council® certified paper.

To my family

ABCDE

Airway. Breathing. Circulation. Disability. Exposure.
This is where it begins. I examine the patient from head
to toe, ensuring first that there is nothing blocking the
airway, that they are breathing. I move along to blood
pressure, heart rate, all the elements of circulation, before
checking their level of consciousness, their blood sugar
and temperature, and finally looking for injury and examining the skin. The one rule of this assessment? To start at
the beginning and only move on once you're satisfied that
each part, the lungs, the heart, the kidneys, is working.

A is always where we start. A. The beginning of the
alphabet. From the Greek, alpha. The biographer and
essayist Plutarch describes how his grandfather referred
to it as the 'simplest sound'. The formation of air in the
mouth and the motion of the lips around the word means
it needs only to be 'gently breathed forth'.

A. The first letter learnt in school, the beginning of
sentence creation, of language, of conversation, of stories
yet to be told. The letter itself shaped with its protective
pointed roof, under which we might stay a while and
think of what more to say. Or cross its connecting bridge
below and move on to the next. Without A, the airway, a
person cannot live.

Whilst studying the roots of medical language at

nursing school, I learnt that the prefix 'a' or 'an' means 'without'. Apathetic: without emotion; amoral: without morality; anaesthesia: a lack of sensation.

For us as nurses, 'A' is both the roof we can stay beneath and the bridge we must cross. If there is a problem with A, the airway, we stay put until we figure out how to fix it. If all is well and the airway is clear, we cross over into B, breathing. But we must start at the beginning.

The anatomy of the airway: the upper respiratory tract – the nasal cavity, pharynx and larynx, which leads to the trachea once its flap of cartilage closes over the oesophagus. Atmospheric air passes through the nose or mouth, is warmed, moistened and filtered and arrives in the lungs in order for gas exchange to take place: oxygen delivered around the body, carbon dioxide sent away in the form of an exhalation. Without a patent airway, a person is unable to breathe. Complete airway obstruction is silent. It may be the quietest way to die.

Airway

Beware the still patient whose chest is silent . . .

University of Leeds, *Recognizing and
Responding to Acute Patient Illness
and Deterioration*

I

The year I left for university, we received a call on the home phone late one evening. Mum picked up. It was my auntie. Her voice was high-pitched and frantic, scrabbling to piece her sentences together like dropped change on the pavement. I listened in. She said that my grandmother's neighbours had been trying to get into her house over in Richmond. They could hear her dachshund barking; he was jumping up and scratching at the window in the living room. I thought of that window, which I'd sat beside over so many years; it stretched from one side of the room to the other, looking out onto the garden. In the garden was the magnolia tree. The flowers were perfectly pink, the petals translucent, lying softly in the grass like shells left behind by the tug of the tide.

After the phone call, the neighbours managed to get inside. They rang us back half an hour later. They had found my grandmother sitting in her armchair, head slumped, the dog nuzzling her feet. She had died.

We drove to her house. Richmond Park was dark. A solitary bicycle light strobed across the grass, catching the retina of a stag, motionless, an unwavering silhouette in the glare.

At the house, Mum asked whether I wanted to see Granny, or would it upset me too much? I told her I wanted to see her and say goodbye. The police were already there. I stood with them in the small kitchen my grandfather had built, whilst my mum went in to see her mother. I stared at the rust on the taps. Mum cried, an after-dark animal sound, clipped short, breath sucked in. It reverberated in the air. I couldn't see her, but I imagined her holding on to my grandmother, her head and hands in her mother's lap. It was the first time I had heard somebody mourn. I kept as still as I could, gripping the edge of the kitchen sink, staring at the rust.

My sister was away, studying midwifery in Stoke-on-Trent. When she came home for the first time, she told me something she had learnt during her lectures on genetics: that women are born with all the eggs they are ever going to have. Thus in some sense, as far back as the day my grandmother was born, she had carried the beginnings of us inside her.

When I went to see Granny in the living room, I found her the same and yet changed. Everything I knew as my grandmother was still there: the gold star of David round her neck, her calf-length pleated skirt, the faint smell of chicken stock and talcum powder, her beautiful silver hair, cut into a bob that curled beneath her chin so that she looked like a girl again. She was the same, but her skin was wax-like and cool and her chest no longer rose and fell with breath. I held her hand and said goodbye.

Five years later, in the summer of 2012, I saw my second dead body when I performed last offices for a patient. She had died on my first placement as a student nurse. It was my first ward, my first morning, my first hour of nurse training. The nursing sister asked me whether I felt comfortable about doing it. I didn't know what to expect, certainly didn't want to say no to anything during my first placement. So Linda, the healthcare assistant, collected what we needed from the store cupboard, and we went into the side room, shutting the door behind us.

Linda was in her fifties, had been working in hospitals for over thirty years. She was nearly six foot tall, broad but gentle and kind. When I'd arrived that morning, I'd asked her if she was the matron. She'd smiled and showed me where the staff room was, and when we sat down to receive the handover, learning about the patients on the ward, she'd nodded at me from across the room, sitting there in the grey stripes of the healthcare assistant uniform. Healthcare assistants carry out numerous tasks in the hospital, ranging from bedmaking to helping to feed, wash and dress patients; they can also gain extra qualifications in blood taking and applying wound dressings. Their presence on the ward is fundamental to a smooth-running shift.

Linda and I barely spoke as we stood on either side of the elderly patient. It is the only time I have washed and shrouded someone without knowing anything about them, without even knowing their name.

The woman was still warm. I wanted to check her pulse but didn't. I didn't know how she had died. All her rings were wedged beneath the gnarled knots of her knuckles, and I wondered how long she'd worn them for. We rolled her and washed her back; she moved easily, having died only an hour before and been left to rest there in the quiet half-light of the room.

Linda took out the shroud from its plastic. It was paper-thin and ruffled at the neck. We took time working out how the woman's arms would be best placed: at her sides, across her chest. We used the material of the shroud to keep them resting loosely across her lap. Linda showed me how to fold the bed sheet, like an envelope, tucking pieces in to keep a foot, a hand safely enclosed. I held my breath when we covered her face. Then Linda went to the far wall, opened the blind and the window. I asked her why she had done that.

She looked at me. 'To let her soul out,' she said.

Linda left the room telling me she would be right back. The room felt small around me, but she soon returned, a purple flower with a delicate furred stalk like a thistle in her hand. She took a safety pin from her pocket and pinned the flower to the top of the sheet. She copied the patient's name and hospital number onto carbon-copy paper and sellotaped it beneath the flower. The last offices complete.

The nursing sister took me to the front of the ward, where the ward clerk's desk was. The TV was on in the day room and I could hear the crowd cheers of the London Olympics winding down the corridor. There were stacks of this week's newspapers and magazines collected in a pile on the desk, alongside scissors and a glue stick.

'I'd like you to spend a few hours helping us to make our Olympic athlete display for the ward,' she said.

I stared at her.

'Here, sit,' she said, and pulled the chair out. 'I'm just up here if you need me.' She nodded and walked back to the nurses' station.

I watched her go, then spent the next half an hour flicking through old newspapers, with no intention of finding athletes to cut up. I looked back at the nurses' station, at healthcare assistants wheeling trolleys of linen into the bays, nurses weaving in and out of bed spaces with trays of intravenous medications and injections. I saw the nursing sister speaking with relatives, making phone calls and writing notes. The ward clerk's desk seemed to drift further away from the rush of the surgical ward. The noise of the crowd roared from the day room, repeats of Olympic gold playing out to the patients passing time watching TV, their legs in casts, propped up on chairs.

In the early days of my nurse training, I felt nursing would never come naturally to me. I was nervous calculating infusion rates, drawing up medication from vials, assisting with sterile procedures and understanding which tasks needed to be prioritized, especially if a patient was deteriorating and time was moving too quickly. I watched everything the qualified nurses did – from making beds to using vacuum-assisted therapy to heal wounds – how they managed to encompass all elements of the role but always made time to stay that little bit longer to make sure their patients felt safe.

I turned back to the ward clerk's desk with the newspapers and magazines laid out in front of me. My mind drifted to the woman in the side room waiting for the

7

porters to come and take her to the mortuary. We were the last people who had seen her. We were the last people who had held her hands. I thought of the flap of the sheet folding over her face, eyes closed, mouth slightly parted, cocooned in a white shroud and a white sheet with a purple flower pinned to the top. The image lingered in front of my cutting and sticking hands for the next two hours.

The nursing sister came to see me.

'Well, you've done an incredible job here!'

I looked down and saw that I had created a sprawling collage of running, jumping, swimming and cycling athletes gathered around the Olympic rings in the centre.

'It's great,' she said. 'Thank you. Now, go and take a tea break and I'll meet you at the nurses' station.'

By the time I got back from my break, the side room was empty. A stripped bed lay in the bright room, bleached mattress gleaming in the sunlight. As I passed, I saw the lime-green flash of the ring-necked parakeets from the park next to the hospital flying by.

I had known this hospital for many years before I came to work in it as a student nurse. It was a new building, opened to much excitement from the local community in 2003, when I was fifteen. It was made of steel and glass, with a second floor that jutted out from the main building on metal stilts, as if preparing for wet weather. Inside, it was bright and airy, the walls decorated with primary-colour flowers and oversized arrows leading the way to the various departments.

It sat at the top of a hill overlooking the village of Farnborough, originally Fearnbiorginga – 'the village among the ferns on the hill'. The surrounding woods were indeed full of lush-leafed ferns, emerald and vein-filled in the summertime sun, brown and crisp at the edges when autumn came.

The new hospital was built on the site of the old Farnborough Hospital, which had been a workhouse in the 1900s but by 1910 had become overcrowded with people suffering from chronic physical and mental health conditions. With the increase of cars on the roads, the number of patients needing X-rays for broken bones and anaesthesia for operations grew. By 1927, the workhouse was now a hospital and had over two hundred beds, the corridors lit by wavering paraffin lamps and the padded cells locked and quiet, barely used.

Operations were carried out in the 'Greenhouse', lit by a gas fire that would be extinguished when anaesthesia was given, due to the combustive nature of the inhaled gas. If not the commonly used chloroform, this may actually have been ether, a volatile liquid that was in regular use as an anaesthetic around this time. Ether, from the Latin *aether*, 'the upper sky', was vaporized and used as a pleasant-smelling gas to send people to sleep.

When I was a child, my dad walked me to school past the hospital on the hill. Down St Thomas Drive, through Sparrow Woods, past the ruins of the half-buried fever hospital, over the stream and alongside the park next to the hospital until we arrived at the school gates. The kids in the playground would ask why it was my grandfather who walked me to school; where were my parents?

Dad was forty-eight when he and my mum had my sister, Daisy, and fifty-one when he had me. By the time he was walking me to school, he was close to sixty. He was tall and broad-backed from a childhood spent swimming, and had a white moustache with a roll-up cigarette always poking out beneath.

In 1947, at the age of ten, Dad was kicking around bomb sites with his friends in Deptford, south-east London, looking for exploded shells, shrapnel, scraps of German parachute often seen fluttering on a fence. He would search for the belongings of the people down his road to give back to them, the ones now living in prefab homes that were bolted together and welded from the outside like cardboard cut-out houses.

At eighteen, he was in the Royal Air Force doing his National Service. He was placed in north Germany as a radar operator, watching a tiny blip on a screen to see if it would creep any closer to their camp overnight. Dad said he lost most of his 20/20 vision on the long nights spent in the green pond-light of the radar room.

Dad was forty-one when he met Mum. He was aware that he was much older than her, and this worried him. Mum too. There was a time when they separated and Mum went on holiday with a man her own age from her theatre company. Spain was cold and loveless, and Mum broke the news to the younger man that she couldn't stay. She came home early and took the train to Fulham, to Dad's house on Archel Road, where she found Dad shelling peas in his tiny overgrown garden. Pink snapdragons grew up against the wall. She sat beside him and helped break the pods, pulling the string down the length of them until the skin separated and the sunlight shone through the green and the peas popped into the bowl.

She told Dad she wanted to spend the rest of her life with him.

Five years later, they had my sister Daisy, and three years after that, they had me. Dad settled in the village among the ferns on the hill, commuting up to town from the station at the bottom. He spent his time reviewing books and films, heaving huge art encyclopedias and crime novels home with him. He stayed up late transcribing warm tape cassettes of Jack Nicholson and Al Pacino interviews onto his memo pad, a roll-up hanging loosely from the side of his mouth, cup of red wine beside him.

On those evenings, I would come downstairs and say goodnight, lay my cheek against his and feel his warm Old Holborn breath on my skin. The feel of my dad's breath on my cheek was always as strong as an imprint.

Later, in nursing school, I would come to know this act, of a cheek held close to lips, as a vital part of assessing a person's ability to draw breath. The feel of breath on the fine, peach-skin hairs of my cheek would tell me if this person were still living; sometimes last breaths become so slow, the only way of catching them is to come in cheek-close and wait for the feel of them.

2

One afternoon Dad came to pick me up from school. We
usually only walked *to* school together. I would walk home
with a friend. There was a storm that afternoon. Dad
wore a long beige trench coat that had been given to him
by a friend whose brother had owned it. This brother had
jumped in front of a train and killed himself. The coat
was dark and heavy from the rain. Dad had belted it
tightly round his waist, pulled the collar up around his
neck and had a flat-peak cap drawn down over his eyes.
He had one hand in his pocket, the other holding the lead
of our three-legged mongrel Ben, who seemed to have
grown smaller in the downpour.

We walked away from the main road and back into the
woods, where we were sheltered from the rain. Dad took
his hat from his head and let Ben off the lead. Ben shook
himself, wagged his tail and hopped further along the
path to drink from the stream. I told Dad that people at
school had asked whether he was my grandad. He didn't
say anything for a while. We walked hand in hand, mine
cold, his warm despite the wet.

'How do you feel about that?' he asked me.

The rain dripped through the gaps in the leaves; I felt a
cold drop creep down the back of my school shirt.

'It doesn't bother me,' I said. '*I* know you're my dad.'

He squeezed my hand and we kept walking through the mud and mulch, watching Ben hop in and out of the river. As we left the woods, Dad took a fern from the wet humus. Crouched by the path, he extracted it with the care of a surgeon removing a clean vein, ready to replant it in a dying limb.

When we got it home, I felt its stalk, furred, soft beneath my fingers. I held it to my cheek. We replanted it, pressing the wet soil around its base. In the mornings, I watched from the living room as Dad, up early in his pyjamas, watered the fern, tending it to make sure its roots could burrow and its leaves could feel the sun; that it could take in the light, allowing it to breathe.

The kids in the playground *had* bothered me. In the days that followed, I would watch Dad cautiously from behind half-open doors, see him picking something off the ground. If I heard him creak or groan, I would pop my head round and check everything was okay. He took tablets for his blood pressure and I would remove them from the cupboard shelf and try to decipher the labels, then place them back exactly as they had been.

3

Before nursing school, I was to have my first experience of being a patient. The park next to the hospital had become a meeting place where I spent my lunch breaks and after-school catch-ups, the boys fighting, girls practising snogging on single-serve boyfriends. We were at the other side of the park, now at the senior school: brown brick and brown glass like a medicine bottle, our uniform brown and yellow. The girls had short skirts, tidemark foundation and peach lipstick; the boys were skinny with stubby ties and always smelt of pickled onion crisps. We'd hang out under the boughs of old oaks, put out cigarettes on the bark, kick bottles in the stream and talk about where we'd go when school was finished with.

I was unwell, and had been for years. During my GCSEs, we read *Lord of the Flies*, William Golding's 1954 novel set against the backdrop of a deserted tropical island. I loved the story but could barely stay awake for lessons. A girl in my class, born prematurely and left with nubs for fingers, stroked my back until I fell asleep with my head in my arms, listening to someone reading aloud. The island in Golding's book was covered in ferns, ferns with light filtering through the fronds, ferns providing green shade or that lay thumped and beaten by the charge of the boys, a tangled place to hide, crouched between darkness and sky.

In my classroom dreams I saw the pale pink curlings of the powerful conch seashell, held high not above the heads of the characters in the book, but above my own, pulling in great swathes of salt-slapped air.

At the beginning of a person's airway, the nose takes in air. Here it is warmed and moistened, easing the flow through the rest of the airway. To help with this process, a long, scroll-shaped swirl of bone widens the surface area. This is the nasal concha, so named for its resemblance to the conch shell. In my island dream, my nostrils flared; I gripped the conch and sucked in breath. I wasn't tired any more, I was awake and alive with the sea raging before me.

Soon it became clear that my sleeping in class was a symptom of a medical problem that needed attention. For as far back as I could remember, I had suffered with swallowing difficulties. In the last years of the condition, about to take my exams, I began losing weight, vomiting in my sleep, regurgitating the meagre scraps I had been able to consume during the day. Mum laundered my bed linen every day, took the curtains down at the week-end to wash away the dark bile I'd sleepily wiped across them in the night.

It took a long time for the condition to be diagnosed. Mental health nurses visited our home trying to gauge whether my vomiting was related to a body dysmorphic disorder, bulimia or depression. I tried to explain that I *wanted* to eat, I *wanted* to feel full and stop the stone-sticking discomfort in my throat, but they avoided eye contact with me and took long notes, casting eyebrow-raised looks at my parents sitting on the other side of the table.

Later, I had frequent trips to the hospital at the top of the hill. I lay strapped to a tilt-table beneath bright strip lights and was instructed to drink a thick, chalky paste disguised as a milkshake in a silver cup. It was hard to swallow and slow-moving, and it sat heavily in my guts.

This procedure is known as a barium meal, a diagnostic test that aims to detect abnormalities in the gastrointestinal system. The weightiness of the meal is not surprising; barium comes from the Greek *barys*, meaning 'heavy'. Through X-ray imaging, the ingested barium glows like a ghostly slug as it travels down the throat and into the stomach and intestinal tract, silvery-white and luminescent on the screen. I watched it myself.

Barium was discovered in the early seventeenth century, when a cobbler from Italy was digging amongst the volcanic rocks of Mount Paderno in Bologna. Here he found what he thought was a precious stone that would make him rich; in actual fact it was barite, a mineral consisting of barium sulphate. He took it home and found that when exposed to light, the milky-white stone glowed for hours, sometimes days. It attracted interest from alchemists across the world and would soon become known as 'the Bologna Stone'.

My barium meal revealed a blockage. The condition was diagnosed as achalasia, a rare gastrointestinal disorder that meant my lower oesophageal sphincter was faulty and wouldn't allow food to enter my stomach. Its cause was unknown. To make the condition worse, I had no peristalsis function: my throat was unable to create normal wave-like muscle contractions to push food into my stomach. Instead, the food would simply back up in the oesophagus until I was sick. At night this became a problem, since my airway was at risk of aspiration: vomit entering the lungs.

At the age of sixteen, I was operated on at the new hospital. Mum came into the anaesthetic room with me and held my hand. I wanted her to stay forever. The anaesthetist told me to count backwards; Mum started to cry and a nurse took her away, then tiredness weighed against me as the thick white propofol travelled through my bloodstream. I was drifting away and soon was asleep.

Some years later, during nurse training, I watched intubation on another patient and thought back to my own on that day. The operating department practitioner tilting my head, lifting my chin, opening my mouth in order for the anaesthetist to look inside with a torch-topped laryngoscope to locate my vocal cords. I thought about my mum. What happened to her when the nurse took her away: where did she go, how long did she cry for?

The laryngoscope is a solid metal instrument with a cylindrical handle and a beak-shaped blade that is put into the sedated mouth, pushing the tongue aside and advancing towards the curtain folds of the vocal cords so that a breathing tube can be inserted into the trachea. The patient is then connected to a ventilator for the duration of the operation, breathing via a machine.

On the day of the surgery to fix my swallowing problem, I was operated on by a seven-foot Iraqi surgeon and his team of experienced Filipino theatre nurses. He performed a Heller's myotomy to cut the taut muscle stopping food from moving into the stomach, and a Nissen fundoplication to stop acid reflux, wrapping my stomach around the oesophagus and stitching it into place. This was done laparoscopically, small incisions and miniature surgical equipment guided by cameras ensuring the operation was minimally invasive. I spent a week in hospital recovering; the five small cuts on my stomach stared up at me like sore, squinting eyes, gradually changing from red to pink as they healed. I asked the doctor if I would have these scars forever.

'They'll fade,' he said.

I felt them in the night; they were hot, and prickled beneath my fingers.

Mum and Dad took turns to stay overnight, but as the week went on, I told them I'd be fine on my own. I put money in the hospital television and watched a late-night horror film in the quiet of my side room: *Sleepy Hollow*, in which the Headless Horseman travels through a small village in New York, murdering its residents by decapitating them.

When it finished, I tried to sleep, pushing the arm attached to the TV against the wall since it wouldn't turn off, the glow from the screen now a fixed square of light against the plaster. I lay there in my bed looking out at the park next to the hospital, at the orbs of light from the bungalows beside the stream floating above the trees.

I closed my eyes and saw a luminous head, lit up from below like a paper lantern, the airway severed so that the head could no longer draw breath. It was completely silent, but blinked at me, eyes wide – desperate, choking eyes – before it disappeared and I finally fell asleep.

Mum and Dad took me home a few days later. My tender stomach felt like a tree root inside me, knotted and twisted, but newly planted, as if it might burst into life the moment I ate something.

Food was no longer a problem. I ate what I liked, things I had missed: bread, crisps, rice, pizza! Anything that I had omitted for the last ten years was now mine. I put on weight and slept well, my cheeks coloured, energy levels swelled, the illness had passed. I thought of the nurse who had stayed with me when my mum left the anaesthetic room. Her name was Star. She held my hand and didn't take her eyes from mine. She told me she would stay with me for the whole operation. I knew I would never forget her. Once I had fully recovered, I completed my exams and went on to do my A levels.

4

In the September after my grandmother died, I went to university. I studied English literature and creative writing at Bath Spa, and spent wet days tramping across campus with my books, staring at the cows lying on their sides in the rain with bellies stretched like drum skins. At night, a crowd of us would travel to Bristol to perform our poetry at open mic nights, or stay closer to home in the kerosene-soaked subterranean bars and cafés of Bath. It was in university halls that I met and fell in love with Rob, who was studying music. Our rooms were three doors apart, mine lit by the twinkle of fairy lights, his by the blue and white streaks of TV against the walls. From the outside our windows looked as if they were performing a nocturnal Morse code through the darkness in between.

In my first year at university I took on a job as a care support worker at Oak Court, a residential home for elderly people with Alzheimer's. I had never looked after people before – I had worked weekends in clothes shops and cafés – but Rob encouraged me to apply and I got the job.

The care home was located in Twerton, a small village to the west of Bath; the locals gave it a twist of the tongue around the 'r'. *Twerrrton*. On one side of the home grew broad-leafed woodland, stretching out into the valley. On the other side lay the white flat-board walls of the estate houses, the Full Moon pub, the Spar and the graveyard, all connected by one long road carved through the centre.

Oak Court stood on a soft grass verge, seemingly always wet from rain. Inside the lobby it was quiet, the carpet freshly hoovered.

On my arrival, I took the lift up to the first floor. As I stepped out, I was met with a loud exclamation: 'THAT'S NOT MY HUSBAND!' An old woman pointed at me from the depths of a sunken armchair and shouted again: 'THAT'S NOT MY HUSBAND!' But this time she laughed, exposing a gummy black hole and a bright pink tongue. Her bald head was smattered with liver spots, wisps of hair orbiting her scalp. She smiled at me, her eyes whirring like Catherine wheels, purple and gold.

This was Sylvia. I would spend many days dancing up the corridors with her, singing 'My Old Man (Said Follow the Van)'. Each time we reached the song's end, we turned to each other, knees bent, slapping our thighs, shouting: 'AND DON'T DILLY DALLY ON THE WAY, HEY HEY!'

Standing there that first morning at Oak Court, I felt stuck to the spot. I wanted so desperately to turn around and leave. The faint smell of ammonia in the carpet, mixed with warm ketchup and buttered toast from the kitchen, was overwhelming. The look of so many paper-thin-skinned elderly people, with bruised legs and heavy-lidded eyes that darted from skirting board to corridor as if searching for somebody to come and take them away, was almost too much to bear. I stood and watched. There was a bathroom door half open and inside I could see a care worker helping an old man off the toilet. As she repositioned his incontinence pad and wiped his bottom, he held on tightly to the sink for balance. Another care worker wheeled a squeaking hoist down the corridor.

''Scuse me!' she said, almost running over my feet. I jumped out the way. The hoist was crane-like and she wore the sling to go with it over her shoulder like a paratrooper.

The exit was nearby but I didn't leave. I put on the blue polo shirt I was given, and worked there for the next two years.

I came to see that in the care home, Sylvia and the other residents could be young again, running through woodland, across disused train tracks, waiting to be asked to dance at the church hall, the boys standing there with wild flowers plucked from Twerton Roundhill in their buttonholes. At other times, they might catch a glimpse of themselves in the mirror as they were now, time dilating so that the curve of the glass brought our two faces – the carer and the cared for – eye to eye: grey hair and false teeth, lipstick and fresh rose blush.

Time didn't stand still at Oak Court. It moved as two children swashbuckling on the stairs would: a step up, now down, a tumble forward, to the side; sit, hold, duck down, lean back. Behind the yellow brick and white plastic-framed windows, time played with its residents and we did our best to make sure they could keep up.

As my time at the home went on, I realized that the old ladies at Oak Court never got sick. There was never any of the chest pain or shortness of breath that I would come to encounter as a nurse. Despite their Alzheimer's disease, these women were made of tough stuff. It was forgetfulness that made them unwell. Forgetfulness that put their airways at risk. When their brains began unlearning the basic functions needed to sustain them, to eat, to breathe. I watched as women I'd sat with talking about the ships coming in and the angels in the garden began to fade away.

Aspiration pneumonia – when food or liquid travels down the windpipe and into the lungs rather than down the oesophagus and into the stomach – is common in people suffering with the late stages of Alzheimer's disease. Whilst I had been aware of the blockage in my throat during my illness, the effect of Alzheimer's on the parts of the brain influencing swallow function meant that dysphagia – swallowing problems – was common for these ladies but not necessarily noticed. Silent aspiration.

There were no more conversations, and Sylvia grew weak from not remembering that food would make her strong, that swallow followed chew. She lay in the soft, eggshell light of her room, somebody sitting with her the whole time. The palliative care nurses came in from the community and taught us how to keep her comfortable: pink sponges to wet her mouth, paraffin balm to moisten her lips, creams to rub onto her skin to keep it intact.

I wasn't with Sylvia when she died. I heard she had half hummed 'My Old Man (Said Follow the Van)', then lay back, tired, waiting for the breeze to take her away.

5

The assessments of airway and breathing are perhaps the most tightly connected of the ABCDE assessments. One leads directly to the other, the mouth and nose opening to the rest of the upper respiratory system, and on towards the lower, where the trachea and bronchi stretch out towards the bellows of the lungs. It is therefore common that in assessing one, the other will naturally be included. If an airway is at risk, clues as to why this could be can be quickly garnered from the assessment of breathing. Whilst it may appear we have moved on, we frequently revert to examining the airway once breathing has shed light on the problem.

As nurses, our exploration of breathing concentrates on the rate, the rhythm, the depth, the oxygen saturations and whether other muscles are being pulled in to assist with the increased work of breathing. Listening to the internal sounds of the body is called auscultation, and is typically carried out with a stethoscope. Auscultating a chest is an advanced way of understanding how air flows through the trachea and the bronchial tree, and provides insight into what underlying disease or condition the patient may have, and what therefore may be affecting the airway.

Listening for breath sounds is a technique first applied

in ancient Greece by the physician Hippocrates. By taking a stethoscope to the patient's chest, all layers of the lung's acoustics can be explored, the inside of the thoracic space brought to life through tracing the ups and downs of pitch, the spikes and softenings of amplitude, and the shades and colours of timbre. A well-trained and experienced ear becomes proficient in understanding the various sounds: the crackles, the wheezes, the high-pitched musical squeeze of stridor, breath sounds emitted by a closing windpipe.

A simple, subtle change in respiratory function can be the first signifier of a patient teetering on the edge of ill health, about to descend into the fast-changing whirlpool of the critically unwell, their airway at risk. It is in this dangerous maelstrom that we as practitioners must retrace our steps: first and foremost, we must protect the airway. At the beginning once more, we listen again, cheek-close, hoping for air. There may be no sound at all; a still patient whose chest is silent is far more frightening than any other sound.

My experience at Oak Court in Bath wouldn't leave me. I often thought of the people I'd looked after. The job had seemed so easy in so many ways. I'd loved it. I missed holding their hands and listening to their stories, being with them just before they went to sleep or in the morning to help them get dressed; meeting their families. When I moved home, I took on a marketing job in the city but didn't enjoy any part of it.

I wondered if I should pursue a career as a nurse. Whilst

doctors do the most incredible things for patients – they inform, diagnose, prescribe, operate, treat and heal – it is the nurses who, despite racking up thousands of steps on their pedometers, are in fact a static constant for the person lying *in extremis* in the hospital bed. In those long shifts it is they who spend hours examining the same patient from head to toe, all aspects of their being uncovered and interpreted in order that we might come to know them better. We learn from each other, and in doing so we become almost fluent in the make-up of the human condition: why we are here in the first place and what we can learn in the time we have.

My sister Daisy was now a qualified midwife and worked at the birth centre in the hospital on the hill where I had been operated on as a teenager. If I were to study to become a nurse, this would be the hospital I would train in, and Daisy and I would be together. I decided to apply for my nurse training.

6

In the months before starting my training, I volunteered with the London Ambulance Service (LAS) to get a better idea of what my new career might be like. A family friend was a high-ranking paramedic in the LAS and was kind enough to let me shadow him for two weeks.

Monday morning, packed lunch and tea flask in my bag, I approached the brutalist grey brick of the LAS HQ in Waterloo, anticipating high-speed blue-lighting across the city. Chris, the paramedic I would be attached to for the next fortnight, was a motorbike responder, working solo, often first on scene. He knew how to drill a hollow needle directly into the bone marrow to provide life-saving fluids when intravenous methods had failed. He assisted medics with roadside thoracotomies, cracking open the chest to deliver cardiac massage, hand-pumping a patient back to life and administering drugs I had only seen on TV: ketamine, tranexamic acid, adrenaline.

Chris and I sat together in the rapid-response car. He had left his bike in the cool brick calm of the HQ.

The call came in: female, 20 per cent burns.

I looked at Chris; he pressed '1' for attending and caught my eye.

'Don't worry.' He grinned at me. 'It's eight a.m.; it's

probably a hot shower or somebody dropped the kettle when they were making a cup of tea.'

We whizzed towards east London, Chris silent, his eyes scanning the road.

As we neared the location, I heard the low-down whirring of a helicopter approaching from behind.

Chris checked his rear-view.

'Hmm,' he said. 'That didn't come in over the radio.'

I looked back, caught a glimpse of the helicopter's blades cutting across the sky, heading towards the park to land.

'HEMS,' he said. The London air ambulance.

We pulled up outside a squat terraced flat on a council estate. The door was wide open; I could see right through into a darkened kitchen.

Chris got out of the car, grabbed kit from the bag and handed me the oxygen cylinder to carry in.

There was a charred smell hanging in the air outside, cloying in my throat.

Chris went in first, and we walked slowly, our rubber soles squeaking on the wet floor.

I glanced up at the ceiling, looking for exposed electricity wires, copper cables, a faulty circuit board. Nothing.

To the right of us was a downstairs bedroom. I peered in and saw an unmade single bed, the covers in a heap at the bottom. The room was empty.

Then we heard screaming.

'Please help us!'

It was coming from the kitchen, the water on the ground deeper here, flickering blue from our car lights outside.

There, naked and white on a stool, was a small creature that looked like a primordial thing, newly born and quivering in the chill.

Chris put his kit down.

'Tell us what happened,' he said to the man who had screamed for help. He was moving frantically from side to side.

He looked younger than me. He wore jogging bottoms and a wrestling t-shirt and his hair stuck out awkwardly on one side. There was a frying pan on the floor by the sink, its innards were star-burst black and the handle glinted with wet.

The naked person on the stool stared straight ahead. For a moment I wondered if they were alive, but I could see the fast flutterings of a heart beneath the thin skin stretched across the sternum. There was barely any flesh on the bones at all.

'It's my mum!' the man screamed. 'You have to help her!'

'Tell us what happened,' Chris said again.

'She was cooking breakfast in the kitchen, and next thing I know the smoke alarm's gone off. I run downstairs and she's on fire! There was flames everywhere, all over her dressing gown, all over her head! She couldn't move, the flames were just eating her up. I chucked water everywhere, all over everything, but I don't know, I don't know if she's breathing now.'

'She's breathing,' Chris said. I could see him eyeing the woman on the stool.

The burnt woman's hands were held open in her lap, the white skin of her arms almost luminous against the burns, thick as rhino hide, yellow at the edges and pink and raw on the inside. There were flakes of blackened skin in a crescent around her.

I had once read in a textbook at school that in the Oro Province of Papua New Guinea, people plaster their skin with clay in a mourning ritual after the death of a loved one. The clay dries, puckers and is scraped off in flakes, a reminder of the loss they have experienced.

The woman's hair was a charred black pompadour. As Chris examined her pupils, he accidentally knocked the quiff of soot and it fell into dust in her lap. The smell was thick and acrid.

I held my shirt up to my face and took deep breaths.

Chris listened to her chest, then beckoned me over. I could barely hear a thing: a half-wind, but mainly a far-stretching expanse of silence. The woman barely moved, as if she was in shock that this had happened to her and the pain hadn't registered yet.

'Let's go,' he said. 'I can't get a line in her here.'

We heard the ambulance pulling up outside.

Chris wanted to give her intravenous fluids to replace the water she would have leaked through the burns. But there were no veins palpable. Instead he wrapped her tightly in cling film to try and stop the burns seeping much more. The amount of fluid inside her body could become so depleted she could go into shock and die.

In the ambulance, the woman continued to stare. The pain must have been agonizing, but she didn't scream. She was breathing, just, but the sound was getting increasingly hoarse, her airway narrowing protectively against the smoke she'd inhaled. Her lips were blue. The other paramedics tried to get a line in her, but her veins were so dry and shut down it proved almost impossible. A baby cannula was eventually put in her foot and warm fluids pushed through.

There wasn't much time. Even untrained, I could see that.

Chris and I ran back to the rapid-response car and said we would meet either the ambulance or HEMS at the hospital. Chris would need to finish the paperwork there.

By the time we arrived, the woman was already in Resus, a department in A&E where patients go who are unstable and could deteriorate quickly. Chris and I hovered outside the blue paper curtains, listening to the familiar scuff of shoes circling the trolley, equipment being ripped from packets, dropped, hooked up, machines turned on.

We heard the team getting ready to intubate her.

'I can't see a thing,' somebody said.

I imagined them looking down her throat with the laryngoscope, the airway too swollen to pass the breathing tube down.

Chris and I looked past each other, listening. The voices became muffled. I imagined everybody hunched over, desperately searching for the space to put the tube.

Chris signalled for us to leave. As we walked outside, he told me the woman would probably be reliant on the breathing machine for a long time in intensive care. That if she did survive and start to get better, he thought they might take her to theatre to surgically create a more permanent airway called a tracheostomy, a hole in her throat with a plastic inner tube keeping it open. This would be a way of weaning her from the life support machine, of keeping her alive as she started to heal.

I didn't see a tracheostomy until many years later, qualified as a nurse and working on a high dependency unit in central London on a night shift. The patient I was looking after was entirely reliant on the incision in his throat to keep him alive: to breathe, for us to suction away secretions and, we hoped, one day to attach a speaking valve to the tube so that he could talk again.

Tracheostomy is one of the most frequently performed procedures on critically unwell patients. It is used to bypass an airway that has been blocked or damaged by traumatic injury, choking, infection, a tumour or, as in this case, severe burns. It can be carried out in an emergency setting, in the forced quiet behind the laryngoscope-lit curtains; or electively, a patient coming to theatre in order to have it done.

Whilst tracheostomies were new to me, they are deep-rooted within medical history and their usage is far-reaching across the globe. It is possible that the ancient Egyptians carved out depictions of tracheostomy procedures on stone slabs as long ago as 3100 BC. In one, a kneeling figure, throat exposed, rests before a seated person directing a pointed instrument towards his neck.

Later, between 2000 and 1000 BC, the Rig Veda, a collection of Sanskrit hymns, poems and scripture, details severed windpipes and life-threatening ligatures in which cut cartilages may provide the solution: a tracheostomy? In this text, a wheel of spinning energy sits at the centre of the throat; flower shaped, it is blue, with sixteen petals tinged smoky purple, and is connected directly to the classical element aether, the upper sky, above the earth, where pure air resides. In medicine, as we have discovered, ether once put patients to sleep, the airway deeply connected to the breath it can draw.

I imagined the woman we brought in lying on the trolley behind the blue curtains. She would be put to sleep in order to have her breathing tube fitted. I thought of where her flower might sit, the purple petals across her throat, her blue lips as she fell asleep, mask applied, sucking in anaesthetic ether, or the pure air from the gods, and then up, up and away, above the hospital, and the Thames, past our island, across deserts and dusty gorges, dreaming of the space above the sky where the light is trapped.

I thought about her son standing in the waterlogged kitchen. I wondered whether he would want to see her this way when he arrived, laid out on the white sheets with her burns staring up at the ceiling, blistered and marbled. In the fresh air outside the emergency department, I took a deep breath.

7

My nurse training began in May. The campus was situated in south-east London. To one side of the Victorian classrooms we had a wide stretch of parkland, a tropical hothouse, and a rose garden connected to the common room. On the other side was the train station, which sent us into central London or the neighbouring hospitals.

In our first year we learnt about anatomy and physiology, the normal functioning of a healthy body, its organs and various connected systems. We learnt about homeostasis, how the body maintains balance, working hard to achieve a stable equilibrium. We learnt how it is able to adapt to extreme environments, producing more oxygen-carrying red blood cells at high altitudes, narrowing blood vessels to conserve heat in freezing climates, developing specialist defence cells to fend off unwanted attack from virus or disease. We learnt how our bodies are in a constant state of flux in order to maintain balance.

For the whole first year of training we were to study health in order that we would better understand sickness when the second year began. At that point, biology would be flipped on its head and we would learn about all the things that can go wrong, the disease processes that gnaw away at healthy tissues, the pathophysiology.

Anatomy and physiology were taught to us from a

cellular level. We learnt about ourselves from the smallest element outwards. Sitting there in the dimmed light of the lecture theatre, we examined the cells of our beings illuminated on the overhead projector.

We were microscopic specks that when observed more closely revealed jelly-filled spaces with suspended parts, filaments of methylene-blue-stained protein lit up from within. Zooming in close, we saw a collection of our pieces, like the intricate workings of a watch counting time. For an hour we gazed at concertina tunnels, wide-eyed lumens, rivulets opening out into wider cavities of fluid, floating globs of protein bobbing on the surface and large bubble-like lakes that destroyed whatever they sucked in. These were the makings of us and I wrote down their alien names in my notebook.

In the classroom we learnt about the spread of infection. We would not be allowed to work on the wards until we understood the fundamentals of infection control and how to protect our patients. The tutor had set up a black metal box with an ultraviolet tray beneath. We were to be taught the hand-washing stages and then have our hands examined beneath the UV light to see what remnants we had not managed to scrub away. Most of the time it was our fingernails, the thin troughs of cuticle lined with debris invisible to the naked eye. And so we did it once more, washing our palms with soap and water, interlacing our fingers, rubbing the backs of our fingers, our thumbs, learning the correct technique and hoping this time we had rinsed it all away.

At the weekend, I was out shopping with Rob. I went

to the shopping centre toilets and realized I was staring at a woman washing her hands, wetting them, lathering soap on the backs, the palms, her fingernails, twisting her thumbs and washing around the wrists as if performing an ancient passed-down ritual. She saw me watching, our eyes meeting in the mirrored glare of the toilets. I blushed, but she smiled and left without saying a word.

Whilst I held all the things I was taught firmly in my mind throughout my training, it wasn't until I was qualified as a registered nurse that I fully understood that minimizing the spread of infection could mean the difference between life and death.

Breathing

. . . every speed swimmer needs a large heart.
Every great swimmer, it should go without saying,
has a heart more powerful and of greater capacity
than that of the average person.

Johnny Weissmuller, *Swimming the
American Crawl*

8

One of my earliest memories is of the breath being taken from me; it appears as clearly and vividly patterned as a phosphene flashing before my eyes. In this memory, the Gorges du Verdon in the south of France stretches out before me; the phosphene flares take on the light of the sun, the river that snakes through the canyon, and the sky, which is blue and cloudless. Me, my sister, Mum and Dad sit laughing and eating a picnic by the water.

Later, Dad and I paddled in the rocky shallows. The canyon is thousands of years old, shaped by ancient streams, and whilst I was small, I felt mighty with my dad walking beside me. Further downstream, banana-coloured kayaks glided across the water, and the smell of pine needles from higher up the gorge drifted towards us.

Dad found a big brown rock and sat, rolling a cigarette and watching with half an eye as I played. I remember wading out further, to the middle of the river. It had looked calm, the current unseen from above the surface, but as soon as I was within its grip, I felt it dragging me down. With one almighty tug it pulled me to the ground, and I felt the rocks beneath the water cut my skin. I could no longer see my dad; the breath was taken from me and I knew I couldn't swim without it. I took great gulps of cold water and felt the force of the river behind me. In that moment, I thought I would be swept away, but in a flash, Dad's strong hands were under my arms and I was plucked from the river, a water-worn pebble grasped for the way its smooth edges held the light.

Despite the water's fierce current in Verdon Gorge, I had always known how to swim. There was never a memory of learning or being taught, but rather a *feeling* that when I submerged myself in the water, I remembered everything. Almost as if the strokes were woven into the fibres of my muscles through our swimming history, practised by my father, my grandfather and his father before him. I found the act automatic, habitual and entirely effortless, if I had the breath to fuel the strokes.

My dad's side of the family had a long lineage of champion swimmers, their photos staring back at me in black and white from the kitchen walls as I ate my breakfast before school. My great-grandfather had been the champion of Ireland, the first to swim the whole of Dublin Bay. His three sons were record-holders in their own right. My grandfather, the policeman Harry Case, brought the crawl to Ireland after teaching himself from the dusty pages of a library book: *Swimming the American Crawl* by Johnny Weissmuller, who, legend had it, had a forehead so vertically sloped that water simply slid right from him. I came to know that Weissmuller died at seventy-nine from pulmonary oedema: water on the lungs.

As a child, I spent most weekends at the local pool with Dad. Up the speed-bumped tarmacked drive we'd walk, with the giant oaks and chestnuts bowing over our heads, heavy with autumn rain, our swim bags slung over our shoulders and the faint smell of chlorine and talcum powder drifting out from within. I took a few lessons as a child but soon quit; my concentration lay in training myself to hold my breath in case the current took me once again.

Whilst my classmates waved various sew-on badges under my nose – gold octopuses and stitch-eyed dolphins holding celebratory streamers that they had obtained for swimming a length or one hundred metres, or perfecting a dive – I was learning how to keep myself absolutely still, submerged at the bottom of the pool, holding my breath for as long as possible. Soon I found that I could swim two lengths underwater without coming up for air. I felt like a magician, capable of great illusory tricks that people on dry land were impressed to see.

As a teenager, just before my operation to correct my swallowing, I went to see the American magician and illusionist David Blaine, who had encased himself in a Perspex box dangling high above the Thames. I stood beneath him and shielded my eyes. The sun was dazzling on the river and bounced off the plastic; people below were momentarily blinded. In the light, it appeared as if one minute Blaine was there, a smudge of dark hair and beard stubble, his sweaty hand splayed against the side of the box; the next he was gone and all we could see were the shining corners of the empty cage and a palm print against the glass.

I read in the news that Blaine had stayed up there, surviving only on water, for forty-four days. He must have been hungrier than me, I thought. He lost 25 per cent of his body weight, and after he emerged, medics studied his physiological response to what he had endured and documented their findings in an American medical journal.

Our bodies are over 50 per cent water, and more than 80 per cent of that water is held in the lungs. The two lungs and the area that houses them can be divided simply into four distinct parts. In the centre are the lungs themselves, described in Henry Gray's *Anatomy of the Human Body* as spongy, elastic and smooth and shiny on their surface; slate grey in colour and able to float in water.

Surrounding each lung we find the visceral pleura, a thin, shimmering layer that follows the contours of each lobe, the fissures and the folds, acting as a caul enclosing the organ. Past the visceral pleura lies a fluid-filled space called the pleural cavity, and beyond this is the parietal pleura, from the Latin *paries*, meaning 'wall', forming a membrane lining that covers the thoracic cavity. The liquid layer in the middle enables the two linings to slide smoothly past each other like plates of glass separated by water during each breath. These four structures – lung, visceral pleura, pleural cavity and parietal pleura – ensure that breathing is as effortless and unseen as possible. We barely notice we're doing it.

A few years later, David Blaine, like me, wanted to see how long he could survive without air underwater. He called this stunt 'Drowned Alive'. In front of a studio audience, he lowered himself into a glowing aquamarine globe of water and closed his eyes. After almost seventeen minutes, the audience gasped and then fell silent as they watched him rise gently to the surface, his head bowed, about to break a world record. Slowly he brought his face above the rim, his skin white and wrinkled as parched earth, his lips cyanosed and quivering. He opened his mouth, taking in air as if it were his first time, dark eyelashes blinking, adjusting to the light like a newborn.

I thought once more of David Blaine during my final year of nurse training. On shift one evening, I watched a man dying, alone on the medical ward. Water was backing up in his lungs and he was gasping for air, stomach muscles in spasm, sucking in breaths as if kicking up from the depths. His lips were blue and he had become confused, wanting only to sleep, his oxygen-deficient blood no longer supplying his brain.

I watched as the patient seemed to disappear.

9

Elm Ward was a large ward with twenty-eight beds. There were many half-rubbed-out marker-penned names on the whiteboard and never enough staff to tend to them all. The ward was meant to be staffed by four nurses and two healthcare assistants on each shift.

The turnover of patients was fast, with people spilling over from A&E waiting to be placed on a ward more suited to their condition. In Farnborough and the surrounding area, the demographic was predominantly elderly. Admissions for broken hips and chest infections were common.

I began my final placement as a student nurse almost two years after the Mid Staffordshire report, a public inquiry into one healthcare trust's thousands of uninvestigated deaths, in which inadequate staffing and negligent nursing were found to be the main causes. Morale among nurses was at an all-time low. There were never enough staff, there was little funding and poor resources, and the depiction of our profession in the media was of demonic and uncaring nurses who had neither the time nor the kindness in their hearts to complete even the most basic of tasks.

Elm Ward was dark and low-ceilinged. The side rooms were mainly used for dying patients, to give them and their families peace and quiet. Eric was admitted overnight to a side room; he didn't have any family with him. He had a chest infection, an exacerbation of his chronic breathing condition, and needed 'offloading' – intravenous medication aimed at reducing the build-up of fluid around the lungs and tissues of patients with heart failure.

Eric had become unable to cope at home; he had stopped washing, eating and taking his heart medication. He was in his late fifties and obese, his hospital gown just covering his lower half. The doctors prescribed diuretics to help him pass the fluid through his urine, but his legs were so swollen that if you pressed a thumb against the surface, an imprint remained. At night he suffered with sleep apnoea, a condition in which he stopped breathing, and so he used a breathing machine overnight to force air into his lungs.

It was hot that day. Eric had kicked off his sheet and lay propped up in bed with his pillows in a V shape; the healthcare assistants knew just the arrangement of pillow origami that would facilitate breathing for these types of patients. It was five o'clock in the afternoon. His eyes were closed and his chest heaved with the exertion of trying to catch a breath. He wore an oxygen mask over his nose, connected to a machine to help him breathe similar to the one he used at home. Known as a NIPPY machine – non-invasive ventilation – this aimed to help him take bigger breaths by blowing extra air into his lungs via the mask and keeping them open for longer at the end of each breath.

Eric was scoring highly on our warning charts and the

doctors had been called. He kept taking the mask off, and when he coughed, I could hear the wet rattle of his lungs. I imagined the branches of his alveoli strung with cobwebs. I talked to him a lot; he didn't reply with words, but instead shrugged his round shoulders or grunted, looking at me for a moment before shutting his eyes to concentrate on breathing again.

The nurse I was working with was looking after seven other patients, the doctor was in Resus, and I had been instructed to take fifteen-minute breathing observations on Eric. I didn't leave the room.

The less he wore his mask, the more confused he became. Once again he grabbed it in his swollen hand and pulled it from his face, resting it on his stomach. Oxygen was no longer circulating to his brain; in just minutes I could see his lips becoming dusky in colour. He was becoming hypoxic. Permanent injury to the brain from lack of oxygen can occur in less than five minutes.

I ran from the room and saw a doctor at the nurses' station. I told him that the man in the side room was dying; that his warning score was fourteen and he was in need of an emergency assessment with possible transfer to intensive care.

The doctor picked up another patient's notes and told me to try and encourage Eric to keep the mask on; to be stern and tell him that he would die if he kept taking it off. He would come and review the patient as soon as he was able. I pleaded with him to come and tell Eric that himself. The thought of re-entering the room on my own was terrifying.

We went in together. Eric threw the mask to the end of the bed. The doctor shrugged his shoulders, telling me and the nurse I was working with that he had the mental capacity to make the decision to remove the mask, even if that decision led to his death. He told me to ring the patient's next of kin to inform them of the situation, and that a DNAR (do not attempt resuscitation) form was already in place from his last admission; Eric had asked for this in case his breathing condition worsened. He didn't want to be put on a life support machine and he didn't want his heart restarted if it stopped.

I looked for a telephone number to ring his family, but he hadn't listed any next of kin or numbers to call. It was now the nurses' job to make him as comfortable as possible, but the doctor would have to prescribe all the symptom-relieving drugs we needed.

I decided to stay with him after that. I left the door ajar, but the noise of the ward had become muted, as if the sound waves were travelling through water. I tried to keep his mask on, my hand pressed firmly against his nose. I told him how sick he would make himself. Eric was still strong; he batted my hands away as I desperately grappled with the mask ties to try and keep it in place.

Finally he spoke. It took me a long time to interpret what he was saying through spasms and gasps, his eyes rolling to the back of his head for seconds of sleep between breaths. He asked me for orange juice. I tried to bargain with him, pleading.

'I will get you as much orange juice as you like if you just keep the mask on,' I said.

He put it on. I checked the settings on the machine to make sure it was working and left the room, relieved that his brain would now be receiving oxygen. I ran to the hospital kitchen at the end of the corridor to fetch the juice.

When I came back in, Eric's mask was resting on his stomach again and he wasn't breathing. I ran from the bedside to call for help, but as I reached the door, he took a breath. I turned around and saw that his eyes were wide, as if he had just remembered how to do it. He asked for the orange juice; I held the tiny plastic carton to his lips and he sucked at it in short, sharp bursts until it was finished.

'More,' he said.

But this time I wouldn't leave him. I tried the mask again. He ripped it off and threw it to the floor.

I started to cry.

In the next moments, Eric began to settle. His body grew still, his breathing erratic; he would go for minutes not taking in any breath at all. Ten minutes passed. Eric could no longer hear me; he didn't open his eyes, his lips were blue-tinged and there was thick, frothy saliva pooling at the corners of his mouth. I wiped it away and pushed the pillows up around his neck to keep his head from lolling. I stroked his sweaty hair back from his face.

Soon no more breaths came. I watched his large, round belly to see if it was working for air, but it was completely still, like the surface of the moon. I looked for the nurse; she was in the side room on the far side of the corridor, dressed in gown, mask and gloves. I asked the ward clerk to ring the doctor; we needed someone to verify the death.

When the nurse came out of the other side room, I signalled for her to come in with me. Whilst we waited for the doctor, we ran warm water in a bowl and put a flannel on Eric's forehead. Later we would wash the rest of his body before wrapping him in a shroud.

After my shift, I went upstairs to where my sister was starting her night shift on the birth centre. I rang the buzzer and was let in. Daisy was in handover, but my tear-streaked face told the support worker on the unit to bring her out for me. I fell into her arms, describing in unintelligible gulps how I had just watched a man die. I told her that he had been alone and that his last breaths had gone almost unheard.

We sat for a long time, the staff room bright with strip lights, the evening becoming dark as the sun set, the smell of day-shift coffee hanging in the air. Daisy held my hand and reminded me that *I* had been there with him, that he *hadn't* died alone. I wasn't family, I told her, I wasn't a friend, somebody he had loved or who had loved him. She wiped my tears.

As I left to let her start her shift, I heard the screams of a woman in the final stages of labour in a nearby room. Then, with my hand on the door, I heard the wet cry of her newborn bringing its head to the brim, breaking the surface.

10

Observing the way a patient breathes is fundamental to spotting the signs of deterioration early. In the middle of the night shift, when the moon has slid behind the silver-rimmed clouds, the slowing of a person's breathing, a longer pause between each breath, may be an indication of something bad to come.

As nurses, we are taught to 'look, listen and feel' all aspects of a person's respiratory system in order to understand what changes might be occurring within the breathing structures. Are there fluids collecting; is there air, solid masses? What sound does the air make as it passes by these abnormalities? What are the breath sounds? Does the chest rise and fall equally on both sides? This person may have a collapsed lung, inflammation of the lung linings, an infection. We bleep the on-call doctor, reassure the patient, apply oxygen, take blood and run it through the analyser; the mobile X-ray scanner wakes the other patients, clattering through the swing doors as the dawn chorus stirs.

The arterial blood we take for the analyser is measured using the numeric scale pH (potential of hydrogen), relating to how many hydrogen ions are present in the solution. This scale gives an indication as to whether the person's blood is becoming acidotic or alkalotic – a normal blood gas would hope to find the pH between 7.35 and 7.45, very slightly alkaline. Battery acid and lemon juice can be scored between 1 and 2, very acidic, whilst soapy water and bleach lead us to the opposite end of the scale, alkaline.

Blood that becomes too acidic reveals that the person may not be breathing out enough of their carbon dioxide, storing the waste product dangerously within their circulation. Their breathing might be laboured; it may be that an underlying disease is inhibiting their normal breathing pattern, or that it is being affected by strong painkilling medication or alcohol. Blood that becomes alkalotic can be caused by a person hyperventilating, breathing out their carbon dioxide at great speed and force like the magician, or the American swimming champion panting at the side of the pool.

The actual atmospheric air we breathe is made up of an unseen mixture of gases and water vapour. Particles lifted from volcanic eruptions, forest fires and sandstorms can contribute to polluting the air, but it is the harmful man-made substances produced by burning fossil fuels, coal and oil that poison it. These invisible but dangerous gases, such as carbon monoxide and nitrogen dioxide, can have a disastrous effect on our lungs, exacerbating chronic conditions, sending us into hospital waiting rooms, changing the pH of our blood and even causing premature death.

The air around us has long been associated with the spiritual world, the word 'spirit' itself deriving from the Latin *spiritus*, meaning 'breath', as if the very air we inhale is not simply gases but is also packed full of demons and deities, ghosts and ghouls. The ancient Egyptians wrote whole sermons on breathing; their funerary text, the Book of

Breathings, provided a handbook to aid the deceased's journey into the afterlife. Centuries later, beneath steaming rainforest canopies, the Mayans believed in the breath soul, the *ch'ulel*, which represented a vital life force able to bind everything in the world together in order to achieve spiritual balance. This life force was often represented as a single jade bead placed in the mouth of the dead to symbolize their breath.

11

The breathlessness Eric had experienced related to heart failure. Heart failure can occur when there has been damage to the heart muscle, leaving it weaker than it was before and less able to pump effectively. This can happen through persistent high blood pressure, inherited cardiac conditions, recreational drug use, heart attack or infection.

Cardiologists diagnose heart failure by studying the patient's symptoms, and through tests such as an echocardiogram, which uses ultrasound to take pictures of the inside of the heart, the valves, ventricles, chambers and vessels. These pictures reveal the size, shape and strength of the heart and, most importantly, calculate what percentage of blood is being pushed out with every heartbeat. When the heart's pump is impaired, it becomes unable to drive blood around the body and the patient can become easily tired and short of breath, their whole body lacking in oxygen.

Depictions of heart failure have existed in medical texts for thousands of years. In China, *The Yellow Emperor's Classic of Internal Medicine*, dated around 2600 BC, linked the tension of the heart to an abnormal accumulation of fluid; in ancient Greece, the Hippocratic corpus described 'bubbling' lungs, heard with an ear pressed to the chest.

The ancient Egyptians were some of the earliest to document the notions of weak hearts and fluid retention. During mummification, the heart was left in the body, which meant that thousands of years later, when mummies travelled through the British Museum's CT scanners in London, the innards of their hearts and surrounding vessels were revealed. Evidence of blockages, known as plaques, told Egyptologists that heart disease was prevalent even thousands of years ago. Evidence of heart failure was harder to find. However, in 2015, a group of researchers were able to identify the oldest known case of the condition by examining the lung remnants of an Egyptian dignitary found inside a broken canopic jar from 3,500 years ago. Here they discovered fluid in the lungs and heart failure cells in the alveoli, only found in people suffering the effects of water on the lungs.

The ancient Egyptians wrote endlessly. From poetry and songs to medical texts and funerary scrolls, their love of language was reflected in the volume of work they left behind. Using their hieroglyphics, historians have been able to interpret and translate reports of early physical examinations conducted by ancient physicians.

The Ebers Papyrus may be one of the best-known of the ancient Egyptian medical texts. Found in 1862 between the legs of a mummy in a tomb in Thebes, it is the longest and most complete of the medical papyri, stretching out for sixty-eight feet. Within its writings, it details a comprehensive insight into the human cardiovascular system, a 'treatise on the heart' that goes on to describe people suffering from fluid overload related to a weakened heart: 'His heart is flooded. This is the liquid of the mouth. His body parts are all together weak.' This could be describing Eric, lying in bed beneath the low ceiling of that hot medical ward, his mouth frothing with pink sputum. It continues: 'When the heart is sad, behold it is the moroseness of the heart, or the vessels of the heart are closed up in so far as they are not recognizable under thy hand. They grow full of air and water.'

Another medical papyrus, translated in the 1930s, sees the Egyptians once again interpreting what appear to be symptoms of heart failure. The Edwin Smith Papyrus works methodically, using a head-to-toe approach to assess a person. It describes the heart as 'too weary to speak', beating 'feebly', with one particular hieroglyph depicting the bluish tinge of cyanosis, indicating the person is no longer receiving enough blood, and thus oxygen, to their body.

Hapi, the god of the River Nile, was pictured in ancient Egyptian paintings as amazonite (or cyanotic) blue, with large breasts and a protruding belly – the fertility of the Nile portrayed through a pregnant stomach, or perhaps a fluid-filled gut overloaded by a weakened heart, the lungs engorged with water from the seasonal flooding of the river.

12

A few years later, qualified as a nurse and working in a busy central London hospital on a cardiothoracic ward, I was looking after a woman called Shui, whose heart was at risk of filling up with water if we did not operate on it. Shui was from China's Guangxi province, in the south of the country; her daughter told us she came from the mountainous karst landscape we might have seen printed on the twenty-yuan note.

Shui had arrived on the ward breathless and clutching at her chest. She didn't speak English, and so her daughter interpreted for her. She told us that her mother felt as if she couldn't breathe, that she was drowning, that her heart felt full to the brim. In Mandarin, Shui's name meant 'water'.

The cardiothoracic surgeons came to see her, and it was decided after investigations and further tests that she would need a cardiac bypass: an operation to divert blood away from the clogged arteries of the heart using a freshly grafted vessel from another limb to re-route the circulation. Over time, the blood flow to Shui's heart had been reduced by her narrowed coronary arteries, meaning the muscle had grown stiff and weak and unable to pump blood as well as it should, contributing to her breathlessness. If she did not have the operation, her symptoms would get progressively worse. She would become tired more easily and her limbs would grow swollen with fluid.

The operation had a high success rate, but it would last at least five hours and would involve Shui's heart being stopped and her lungs deflated. A heart-lung machine would take over the job of beating and breathing for her. There might be three surgeons or more working on her at the same time, two of them tackling the heart in the thoracic cavity, another stripping a vessel from her leg to use as a graft around the heart.

The information was relayed to Shui via her daughter. They spoke for a long time to each other in Mandarin. Shui held her chest and panted for breath, her brow furrowed, shaking her head as if to say she couldn't take any more. She consented to the operation and would be brought down early the following morning.

It was my task to prepare Shui for theatre overnight. The procedures were explained to her by her daughter, and whilst she looked frightened, she smiled and held our hands as we talked. I helped her to wash with the luminous pink antimicrobial soap needed for theatre, then shaved her arms, legs, chest and groin, took her blood and ran an ECG. When the clock struck midnight, I removed her water jug; she was to be nil by mouth until the porters came to collect her in the morning.

During the surgical checklist, I asked whether Shui had any metalwork in her body, any prosthetics or loose teeth. She listened to her daughter's translation and then nodded. I reassured her that we would keep her dentures safe in a pot for when she came back out of theatre. I asked her if she had any jewellery on, and she lifted her wrist, a jade bracelet gleaming in the gloom.

It was beautiful, like ocean-smoothed rock, the colour of green sea foam. The daughter told me that her mother had received it on her wedding day fifty years ago and kept it on ever since. There was no clasp to be unhooked; it was one smooth, hard loop of stone that wouldn't come off.

By now it was late and I didn't want to call the doctor about the bracelet. I decided that we should let Shui sleep, propping her upright in the bed in the hope that she would get some rest before the operation.

In the morning, the porters came and we loaded the bed up with her medical notes, charts and printed blood reports. Shui looked tiny tucked beneath the sheets. I checked her identity wristbands; the jade bracelet still lay cool and intact against her skin.

Outside theatre, the brakes were put on the bed and I held Shui's hand as we waited for her to be checked in by theatre staff. She didn't look frightened any more. When the theatre nurse came, I passed him the medical notes and Shui softly rubbed the jade bracelet beneath her fingers.

As he ran through the checklist, the theatre nurse noticed the bracelet. I told him it wouldn't come off. He jogged away through the automatic doors to find the surgeons.

He was back within seconds.

'It has to come off,' he said. 'When the anaesthetist puts in the arterial line, her wrist might swell, or they may need the vessels in that arm for harvesting.'

I nodded. 'It really won't come off,' I said.

The theatre nurse looked cross. He sent a porter to

A&E to get some wire cutters, and they arrived within minutes, packed in a cold steel briefcase. A&E were used to receiving trauma patients requiring the use of the tools to remove impaled objects, broken machinery or metal-work from injured limbs.

Shui looked frightened now, as more people came out to see what was going on. The theatre nurse went to find a Mandarin-speaking member of the team, and he arrived at Shui's bedside clutching the wire-cutter briefcase and speaking quickly: the operation was already delayed, the consultant was scrubbed and ready to go.

Eventually Shui nodded and was handed a piece of paper to sign.

'What did she say?' I asked. 'Are you sure she agreed?'

The staff member looked towards the doors of the operating theatre.

'She says she wants the operation, she wants her breath back, and will consent to us removing the bracelet in any way we can.'

Shui held her wrist tightly in the bed.

The man tapped the wire-cutter briefcase with his pen.

'But she'll only let us cut it off once she's asleep.' He smiled and walked quickly back into theatre, his surgical gown flapping like coat tails behind him.

13

I met Michael a few months later. I had been qualified for one year, and whilst I was still in the same cardiothoracic specialty, I worked most of my shifts on the neighbouring high dependency unit (HDU), where patients went after their cardiac surgery.

Michael was a small man, the height of most of the nurses, quite different from many of the other male patients on the ward, who stooped to collect their tablets from us. They were tall men with wind-swept white hair and broad shoulders from days spent lifting the canopies on RAF aircraft or lugging heavy National Service-issue kit. Many of these patients had done their National Service in the 1940s and 50s, and often talked to each other about their memories of that time. More than one in eight people over the age of seventy-five has some form of heart valve disease.

Michael was too young for this. He had been a fire-fighter, retiring just a few months earlier at the age of fifty-five after thirty years of service. He and his wife had one teenage daughter and were planning their retirement together. They had booked a big trip to celebrate; they wanted to see Asia and had bought a round-the-world ticket. Soon after retiring, however, he had had a major

60

stroke that left him with left-sided weakness and aphasia: he was unable to speak at all.

To order his meals from the ward hostess, he pointed at a laminated pictorial menu, and she soon learnt to give him yes/no-answer questions: 'Do you want orange juice with that?' 'Do you want a dessert?' Communication became bare and transactional, language stripped to skeletal branches too weak to support the weight of words once ripe with colour.

Michael had been in neuro rehabilitation at his local hospital since the stroke and was engaging well with therapy and making progress; the idea of some sort of holiday was not entirely ruled out yet. During his time in rehabilitation, he had had investigations to determine the cause of the stroke. The cardiac team found an infected heart valve, and he had been admitted from his local hospital to ours in central London for a heart valve replacement.

His wife told some of the nurses that he had been senior in the fire brigade; that she couldn't believe that the man who had dragged blanketed bodies out of poker-hot blazes was now himself shrouded in thin hospital blankets to beat the draught.

My colleague Caroline was one of the only nurses able to understand Michael. To most, his silence and expressions were indeterminable, and when – quite understandably – he became frustrated at the miscommunication, he would stare unblinking and yellow-rimmed at whoever had failed to get the message. Caroline's presence on shift became vital for the healthcare staff, the nurses, the doctors, and for Michael himself. She was a clear stream. With her around, the water grew calm, no longer murky. Clarity and comprehension were close, undisturbed by the rocks and rough meanderings of wrong words and unmoored meaning.

One night shift, I was working on the cardiothoracic HDU next to the ward. A different colleague was looking after Michael. I was busy in the side rooms with a patient requiring high doses of a blood pressure infusion and a patient on four-hourly intravenous antibiotics when I became aware of the glow from Michael's bedside light, still switched on in the early hours, and a figure sitting upright at the edge of the bed.

It was Michael's first night after his operation, day zero as we call it. This meant that he was still attached to numerous illuminated infusions to support his organ function, pain levels and hydration status, bags of fluid backlit by pumps, midnight ships blinking through the night. In his post-operative state, and with the disorientation that arrives as darkness falls, he had become delirious, tugging at the IVs in his neck, the arterial line in his wrist, the chest drains and urinary catheter, unable to understand why we were keeping him captive in the bed. In fact, we hardly ever keep a patient in the bed; it is more dangerous to do so, and using the rails as restriction can be deemed as mechanical restraint.

It is common for patients to become confused after an operation. Often the effects of the anaesthetic drug take a while to subside, but patients who have spent time on the heart-lung machine during surgery can also experience a strange out-of-body delirium, colloquially known in the specialty as 'pump-head syndrome'.

Michael was small, but nearly always with delirium, especially at night, comes strength. On one night shift I saw a little old man try and throw himself through a window, so convinced was he that we were Russians spying on him whilst he worked on the railway overnight. With the help of two healthcare assistants, three nurses and the doctor on call, we were able to get him back into his bed. He was exhausted after trying to escape the ward all evening, and eventually fell asleep, with somebody sitting beside him for the rest of the night to make sure he didn't hurt himself.

One young woman I looked after on the unit, whose brain had not received enough oxygen during her heart attack, accused me of soliciting her young children on the internet. She told this story to the oncoming day shift, including my manager, and held up blank tabs on her smartphone to try and emphasize her point. I'm sure her own reality was terrifying that night.

On this particular night shift, if Michael began pulling out lines, he would put himself at risk not only of haemorrhage but also of air embolus, an air bubble travelling through the IV-less hole in his neck towards his heart or brain, where it could cause a heart attack or another stroke.

As a last resort, we use medication to subdue patients: haloperidol, which between ourselves we call vitamin H. We use it rarely in cardiac patients, however, as it causes too many other symptoms: dangerous rhythms that alter the electrical conduction of the already fragile heart. There are so many other ways of reasoning with and calming a patient, and amongst us nurses, the intramuscularly administered vitamin H is thought to actually exacerbate confusion. This medication is not routinely prescribed and therefore we cannot give it until we have spoken with the doctor, who similarly agrees it is in the patient's best interests to administer it. However, if we disturbed the night registrar every time we had a confused post-operative patient, the on-call doctor would never get any rest.

Most of the time a patient who feels confused needs to be listened to, to some extent agreed with and then respectfully but skilfully delayed or distracted in some way. Communication is paramount. On these occasions, we sit down and agree with the person that yes, they *may* be late for work, their wife *may* be waiting, it *might* be too expensive to stay here any longer, then assure them that a phone call will be made to work, wife or institution to confirm that this change of plan is all in hand and everybody is agreeable to it.

This kind of confusion often works in cycles: for an hour the patient will retain the plan and lie quietly in bed, the infusions will remain unblocked, the heart monitor uninterrupted; but soon the process will start again, the delirium rising like a skin blush, and so the script will continue for the next ten hours.

Often shifts like these, which host a severely delirious patient, finish in the morning with the other nine patients on the ward looking chalky-mouthed and red-eyed. They too have been up all night, calling across the room for the patient to 'Relax!' 'Hang in there!' or just 'Shut up!' The day staff walk onto the unit, out of breath from cycling to work,

Lycra-clad and smelling of roasted coffee, and feel the uneven splintered deck from the night before rocking beneath their trainers. I once came on shift to find a chair lying in the centre of the room, broken into bits, as if lightning had struck it overnight, and a bird-nest-haired, sweaty-browed night nurse desperately trying to remove its remains. I never found out what had happened.

That night, Michael and the nurses bore the brunt of the storm and we were all safe. The night nurse had stayed beside him, reassuring him that when the morning came, his wife would be back to see him, and finally he had fallen asleep in the early hours.

After that night shift, Michael returned to his normal self; however, his oxygen saturation levels remained lower than average, an occasional symptom after cardiothoracic surgery, the lungs needing time to re-inflate. Despite his breathing rate being normal and showing no increased effort, he soon required the critical-care nurses to set up a bedside machine called Optiflow. This consists of a hydrated nasal cannula, which pushes hot high-flow oxygen into the lungs, and is able to be worn relatively comfort-ably by the patient via a head strap and small tubes up the nose. The machine improved Michael's numbers and his arterial blood gases, but as soon as we trialled him with-out it, everything fell once again.

His stay on the HDU was dragging on. Other patients soon followed the usual post-operative trajectory and were stepped down to the main ward and then cheerily discharged home. Michael, on the other hand, had another chest X-ray to try and determine why his lungs were not working as they should be. There were no changes evident – no new infection or lung collapse, both reasons as to why he might have poor gas exchange. Even so, he was treated with another course of intravenous antibiotics just in case something else was brewing, and was moved to the main ward through the porthole doors, where he could mobilize more freely. The doctors hoped that if he was able to walk about more, it might help shift any remaining fluid around the lungs.

When she was on shift, Caroline would check in with Michael every couple of hours, despite having her own post-operative patients on the HDU. If his wife wasn't there, she would make sure Michael had everything he needed; the other nurses were simply too busy with their own patients to take the time to try and interpret his eyebrow raises and hand gestures. On her break, she would go to the coffee shop and bring him a chocolate milkshake.

A few days later, I was back on shift and Michael was with us once again on the HDU. I saw a newly inserted stringy-looking chest drain hanging from his side and the Optiflow machine once again flashing next to the bed. His eyes tracked me as I walked to the staff room to get changed; they were still yellowish, owl eyes that had seen more of the night than any other patient.

'What happened?' I asked the nurse in charge from the shift before.

'Pleural effusion,' she said. 'Poor guy, he came back in overnight.'

Pleural effusion meaning water around the lungs that needed to be drained.

66

'Hopefully the drain will sort him out once and for all,' I said. 'It would be great to get him home soon.'

The night nurse nodded.

Later that day, Michael's local hospital rang us and said that they were giving his rehabilitation space to another patient; his inpatient stay with us had gone on so long they could no longer hold it for him. The stroke rehab was vital for Michael to regain his previous quality of life: football training with his daughter, travelling around the world with his wife. He was a relatively young man; he might still have thirty more years of life within him, maybe grandchildren to watch grow up.

All the doctors were keen to get him home. At morning discharge planning, soft pressure with added smiles was put on the nurses to get him up and about more regularly so that the fluid would drain and he could be repatriated back to the local hospital, rehab, and home where he belonged. Michael stared past the doctors during the ward round, his face lopsided from the stroke, lips pursed as if about to form a word.

Once more he was stepped down to the ward, but a week later he was back in the HDU. His breathing had got worse, the muscles in his stomach rapidly sucking in breath to assist his lungs, along with poor oxygen saturations. More chest X-rays were ordered, with a comprehensive review from critical care, but no changes were seen and there was no need this time for a chest drain to be inserted.

Michael looked tired. He spent more time resting on the bed, he had lost weight and his face was grey. We were pleased to see that he was still wearing his own clothes, jeans and a T-shirt; the hospital gowns shrink patients, and anonymize them too. His wife brought in clean clothes every other day, and the sight of a new outfit folded perfectly at the end of his bed like a Christmas-morning stocking was almost unbearable to witness.

His wife sat beside him in the oversized bedside chair and read the paper to him; his daughter showed him photos from her latest Saturday football match. They had another dad running the line these days. When he smiled, the left side of his mouth curled upwards as it should. It was the first time I had seen how his face might have looked before the stroke.

Since the cardiothoracic doctors had had Michael under their care for nearly three months, they thought it best to consult other teams to find out if there was any other reason why Michael simply couldn't catch his breath. The respiratory team ordered a bronchoscopy – an invasive procedure that involves a fine-bore tube being inserted into the lungs to look for any abnormalities.

Afterwards, Michael came back to the ward with a sore throat and groggy from sedation. Caroline took her break and bought him a chocolate milkshake. He slurped the whole thing, then kissed her hand. His wife laughed, then cried through a smile and laid her head on the pillow next to his as he drifted off to sleep.

From his charts, it seemed he had put on a few pounds, but his skin was still grey, mottled beneath the surface like the beginnings of a storm. His eyes were no longer yellow, but amber now.

After the bronchoscopy, the respiratory consultants

ordered yet another chest X-ray, and the next morning a whole new team arrived on the ward. We didn't recognize them. This was a big team, with medical students and junior doctors in tow, probably keen to find an exciting case to discuss. They hadn't been to this ward before and asked the healthcare assistants where Bed 11 was. The assistants pointed the way, hot meal trays balanced on their arms.

I watched the students hovering at the nurses' station whilst the consultant and the registrar went to Michael's bedside, where they pulled the curtain around. Caroline told me later what had transpired. Apparently Michael's breathing hadn't improved because he had pulmonary fibrosis. This meant that his lungs were thickened and scarred. The medical team weren't sure what the cause was; his job in the fire service may have contributed, but equally, the cause of the condition might never be found. They suggested that the infection in his heart valve might have made the condition worse, but they couldn't be sure. They didn't know how long his lungs had been damaged, but they were sure they had deteriorated significantly over the last few weeks. They said the scarring would have been present when he had the stroke, but the doctors then were quite rightly occupied in treating the stroke, then the cardiac problems, and thus it had deteriorated beneath the surface for many months without detection.

The team spoke to Michael and his wife over the next couple of days. They explained that the fibrosis and Michael's breathing had become so bad that whilst medication might prolong life, it would only be by a few weeks;

a month at most. Michael accepted this, although his mind was often elsewhere and he would get up frequently to sit somewhere else during the discussions. The doctors wondered if the infection had perhaps now spread to parts of his brain. His breathing was short and clipped; it was difficult for air to pass through the thickened tissue around the air sacs in his lungs. His condition was worsening at a rapid rate; every time he pursed his lips to blow out air, a dry cough came first, the sound weak and raspy.

He was moved in a wheelchair to a respiratory ward that was more suited to his current condition. Caroline cradled his notes and walked beside his wife, a porter pushing him along whistling an old Nat King Cole song. She took over an hour to return to the HDU, so comprehensive was her handover. She wanted the nurses on the respiratory ward to feel like they too knew Michael and could understand what he might want or need in his last weeks.

It turned out it was his last day. That night, his breathing deteriorated again. The family and medical team had decided that if he were to have a respiratory and subsequent cardiac arrest, he would not be resuscitated. The chances of him surviving a cardiac arrest in hospital were poor, due to his frail condition, and if he were resuscitated and survived, he might wake up more unwell than he had been before, since oxygen would not have been travelling to his brain or other organs whilst his heart had stopped.

In the notes, we read that the palliative team had been by his side, setting up a syringe driver to ease his symptoms, drip-feeding a sedative, a painkiller and a secretion inhibitor beneath his skin to make his final breaths less laboured.

He died in the early hours, his wife and daughter by his side. A single entry from the junior doctor read: *Death certification performed, nil heart sounds, pupils fixed and dilated, RIP Michael.*

I thought of his wife and daughter's journey home, the turn of their key, stepping through the front door, seeing that the flat was the same but realizing that everything had changed.

After a couple of months, we received a card from his wife. It told us that her daughter had passed all her A-level exams and they were off round the world together, to Asia and beyond. At the bottom she wrote that they would 'cheers' every sunset beer to Michael, loving husband and father, always.

14

Before I qualified as a nurse, I had to undertake mental health training. During the first year at nursing school I was to spend two weeks at Brookfield Park, an inpatient mental health unit in Farnborough with three adult wards. My only experience with mental health was from my time spent at the care home in Bath, where I had looked after elderly people with Alzheimer's. The sun had shone through the windows and the bedrooms had smelt of freshly cut flowers and talcum powder. And whilst there had been sadness, in the lives that had once been and the stories no longer remembered, there was always laughter and the sound of a half-finished old tune drifting down the corridor before lunch.

I didn't know Brookfield Park but had walked past it many times on my way to the main hospital. It sat next to the car park, a squat, flat-roofed building with bricks that were hard to tell the colour of since police cars were always pulling up outside, flashing their blue against the walls.

At Brookfield Park I was placed on Davidson Ward, an acute psychiatric unit for people aged between eighteen and sixty-five. It had a two-door system that locked you in between each door, keeping you encased behind glass before the next one opened. There were CCTV cameras in the corners of the rooms, and each bedroom had an emergency alarm that glowed orange overnight.

I met Ahmed on my first day at Brookfield Park. He had an appointment with Dr Bauer, the Austrian psychiatrist who came on Wednesday mornings. Dr Bauer had round brass-rimmed glasses that he wore halfway down his nose, and his hair was white-blonde and slicked over to one side. I sat quietly at the back of the room; as a student nurse, I was invisible.

There was a knock on the door and Dr Bauer called, 'Come in.' A slight pause, and then a tall man – he must have been well over six foot – entered, his trainers padding softly on the carpet. He wore a black Islamic thobe and a black cotton kufi hat with crocheted holes like a child's paper snowflake. He tucked his long robe neatly behind him before he sat in the chair, and lowered his eyes to the ground, waiting for the psychiatrist to speak.

Dr Bauer leant back in his chair; it creaked loudly. He crossed his legs and opened a notepad, twiddling a thick gold pen between his fingers.

'Mr Mohammed,' he said, as if announcing to somebody else in the room that Ahmed had arrived.

He wasn't talking to *me*; I was a student nurse, invisible.

'Tell me . . .' His voice was dull against the flat-board walls and the thin carpet. I could feel the floorboards beneath my shoes. 'Your parents brought you here: now why was that?'

Ahmed looked up, his long fingers interlaced before him. His face was calm, voice low.

73

'I haven't been well,' he said. He didn't look at me; I wondered if he even knew I was there.

'Go on,' Dr Bauer said, gesticulating with his hand.

'I was working in Tesco . . .' Ahmed lifted the sole of his trainer from the carpet; he glanced at the underside for a moment and then back to Dr Bauer.

Dr Bauer waved his hand again, encouraging Ahmed to speak. He recrossed his legs, moved the gold pen to the other hand.

'I was getting funny phone calls, late at night.'

'Somebody you knew, Mr Mohammed?'

'Nah,' Ahmed said. 'There weren't nobody there. It was always dead quiet. But then I started *making* calls. My phone would just dial the number right in front of me and I'd have to listen.'

'And what would you hear?'

Ahmed looked up to the coving, his eyes resting there whilst he pondered.

'At first I thought it was Arabic. But like Arabic sped up, or underwater, all gibberish and fast like.'

'Could you understand it?'

Ahmed shook his head, then ran his thumb and forefinger over his beard.

'Not at first,' he replied. 'Like I said, it was kind of Arabic but then just . . . rubbish. One time I hung up the phone but it rang straight back, and when I listened that time, I could understand it.'

'And what did it say, Mr Mohammed?' Dr Bauer tapped his pen against his notepad. Ahmed looked at the pen.

'It was angry that time. It told me I needed to kill my

family and then myself. It said it were an angel sent to tell me, but . . .'

Dr Bauer waited. Ahmed's wide eyes looked up to the ceiling again.

'But?' Dr Bauer said.

'But I know now it weren't an angel. It told me it were made from the light, but really it came from the fire.'

I sat motionless, anxious not to disrupt Ahmed's story.

'How long have you worked at Tesco, Mr Mohammed?'

Ahmed smiled slightly.

'Four years, but I'm quitting now. I want to go to university. I've saved some money.'

'I see.'

The room was quiet whilst Dr Bauer wrote notes on his pad. Ahmed was unmoving in his chair, his hands locked together in his lap.

'Why did your parents bring you to us here, Mr Mohammed?'

'Because of the jinn,' he said.

'Jinn?' Dr Bauer repeated.

'The thing on the phone that I thought was an angel but all along it was a jinn. It tried to trick me and I didn't know at the time. My parents guessed before me; that's why they brought me here.'

'Correct me if I'm wrong, but if your parents thought it was a jinn, why would they bring you to me, Mr Mohammed? Why wouldn't they take you to your local imam?'

Ahmed frowned and shuffled his trainers in front of him. He looked at Dr Bauer, then shrugged.

'Are you convinced that you really were speaking on

the phone to a jinn, or could there be something else going on in your mind?'

'Like what?' Ahmed said quickly.

'How are you finding the medication we're giving you?' Dr Bauer said, eyes on his pad. 'Is that helping, or are you still receiving phone calls?'

Ahmed shook his head. 'Nah. But I've only just got my phone back anyway.'

'Good. Let's keep the medication going then. And your parents? Will they come in and see you?'

Ahmed shrugged again; he was no longer looking at Dr Bauer.

'Okay, Mr Mohammed, that's enough for today. I'll see you again next week.'

Ahmed dusted his lap and stood up, head lowered. He closed the door softly behind him as he left.

'Well!' Dr Bauer said, spinning round to face me and slapping his thigh loudly so that I sat up in my chair. 'I've not had possession in a while! And no insight at all.'

I raised my eyebrows. 'What is a jinn?' I asked. 'Is it some sort of spirit?'

'Yes,' Dr Bauer said. 'It gets quite complicated, the line between spiritual belief and mental disorder, exorcists and psychiatrists. Mr Mohammed is clearly delusional; his positive response to the medication we're giving him is evidence of that. As you can see, though, he still clearly believes he has been possessed by this jinn.'

'What is it like?' I said. 'The jinn?'

'Well, I've read a few papers on it.' Dr Bauer looked away. 'The Quran describes it as a spirit that walks on the earth as we do, only it is invisible to us, completely unseen. You heard Mr Mohammed talk of angels and light; well, these jinn spirits are apparently born from smokeless fire.'

I nodded, imagining Ahmed in his room after work talking on the phone to the unseen spirit.

'I'm going to get a coffee,' Dr Bauer said, and he slipped his notepad and gold pen into his jacket pocket and left the room.

It was quiet when he'd gone. If I listened hard enough, I could just about hear the *chhhk* of lighters in the court-yard, the flick of thumbs and the small metal wheel sparking a flame.

There was something frightening about a smokeless fire, about something so dangerous occurring with noth-ing to warn of its arrival.

15

A fever is classified as a temperature over 37.5° Celsius. During a high temperature, a substance is released into the bloodstream that raises the set point of the brain's internal thermostat. This heat-generating substance is called a pyrogen, from the Greek *pyr*, meaning 'fire'.

In the summer of 1948, New York was experiencing a heatwave. Residents flocked to nearby beaches or submerged themselves in the city's fountains. The temperature rose to 42°C and authorities opened up the fire hydrants to let people cool off in the streets. At the hospitals, children were brought to emergency departments sweaty and prostrated, lying limp as leaves in their mothers' arms.

The clinical presentation of these children in the sidewalk-fried summer of the late forties led to a groundbreaking scientific discovery in the ensuing years. The sweat of these sun-struck New York infants was found to have a high salt content and led the way for further developments in the classification of cystic fibrosis, such as sweat testing to aid a diagnosis.

New York in the forties was not, however, the first time CF had been noted. In the eighteenth century, a German medical text wrote of the 'bewitched' and 'cursed' infant that tasted salty, and a nineteenth-century *Almanac of Children's Songs and Games* declared that 'the child will soon die whose brow tastes salty when kissed'. Testing sweat for salt content is still a well-used form of diagnosing the disease, along with other investigations.

I was over a year qualified and still working on the cardiothoracic HDU in central London. Shannon arrived late one evening, flown in by helicopter from the north of the city. She was wet with salt-streaked sweat, barrel-chested and coughing, breathing with flotsam lungs that let the water in. She had suffered a blunt-force trauma to her chest, a physical assault that had left her collapsed in a stairwell with rib fractures penetrating her left lung. She required immediate cardiothoracic intervention. When she arrived, her past medical history was relayed and it transpired she also had cystic fibrosis (CF). She was twenty-three years old, one hundred and sixty centimetres tall, and weighed just thirty kilograms, categorized as 'severely underweight' on the body mass index scale.

Shannon was rushed to theatre, where a chest drain was inserted into her pleural cavity, the slippery space between the lining of her lung and her chest wall. The rib fracture had pierced the surface of her left lobe and resulted in air leaking into the surrounding space. This excess air altered the pressure inside from its normal functioning, putting extra strain on the lung and causing it to collapse.

In theatre, Shannon was breathing with just one lung, which was already damaged from chronic infections relating to her CF. The surgeons needed to relieve the pressure around her collapsed lung; failure to do so could put her at risk of going into respiratory arrest, unable to breathe by herself any more.

The surgeons quickly anaesthetized the area and inserted a chest drain – a tube attached to an external bottle filled with water, which is in turn attached to a suction unit – finally allowing the air to escape and the lung to gradually re-expand. Shannon was then moved to us on the HDU, where we could look after her.

The next morning I received handover and was allocated Shannon to look after for the shift. At eight a.m., she was asleep in bed. Shannon looked like a child herself, though she was twenty-three years old, dressed in Dalmatian pyjamas, her hair tied messily back from her pale face with a sequinned scrunchie. She had one hand resting lifelessly above her head and her forehead was glistening with sweat despite the coolness of the room.

Shannon was small for her age because of her condition. Cystic fibrosis is a genetic disorder dominated by thick, sticky secretions that inhibit both growth and respiratory function. In healthy people, the CFTR gene (cystic fibrosis transmembrane conductance regulator) pumps chloride into our secretions in order to draw water towards them, thinning the mucus to aid normal breathing. In cystic fibrosis sufferers, however, the CFTR gene is defective and unable to do this, resulting in a build-up of mucus.

People with CF primarily experience malabsorption, the secretions stopping digestive enzymes from breaking down fats and proteins, resulting in poor nutrition and failure to thrive. Chronic chest infections develop in the lungs due to a build-up of mucus that can lead to bacteria becoming a permanent resident within them, not necessarily causing symptoms each time, but rather lying dormant, a shadow waiting in the wings.

Often symptoms do present and the person will need to be admitted to hospital to receive intravenous antibiotics. The infection becomes difficult to treat when bacteria develop resistance to the antibiotics we use. Pseudomonas aeruginosa is one particular bacterial infection that commonly affects people with CF. This bacterium is able to withstand harsh environments, and is usually found within stagnant water sources and soil. On infected sputum it often smells sweet but rancid, like gone-off milk or rubbish left too long in the sun. Pseudomonas bacteria are opportunists, travelling from unwashed healthcare workers' hands or hospital equipment to lungs and immune systems already weakened by disease. Thus, those with CF are at high risk of becoming infected.

I let Shannon sleep and recorded her observations from the monitor above her bed onto the chart. Her breathing was within normal ranges, oxygen saturations good, but her breaths were shallow, as if she couldn't quite fill her lungs to their depths. In the gloom I shone a pen torch at the chest drain bottle and tubing, which swung each time she breathed, but the fluid inside didn't bubble, which might indicate a leak in the drainage system. It had drained twenty-five millilitres of fluid since the night nurse had checked. I recorded it on the chart. I checked the suction at the wall and closed the door quietly; she had had a long night with little sleep, and I would wake her up when her medications were due.

When I next went in, Shannon was sitting up in bed, illuminated by the screen of her phone.

'Police been on the phone,' she said as I came in. 'They've got 'im in custody.'

'Shannon, I'm Molly,' I said. 'I'm going to look after you today.'

Shannon's thumb scrolled down the screen; she didn't look up at me.

'How're you feeling?'

'Fuckin' 'urts,' she said.

'I'm sure. Chest drains aren't pleasant.' I smiled. 'You've done very well to get any sleep with it in. Do you want some painkillers?'

She nodded, still looking at the phone. 'But none of that paracetamol crap, just the morphine.'

'That's fine,' I said. 'I'll look at your prescription.'

I clicked on the drug chart and saw endless medication relating to Shannon's CF. She had big capsules of vitamin supplements and pancreatic enzyme replacements. Alongside them were inhalers and mucus suppressants to work on the lungs. She was fluent in her medication list; she knew what she wanted and what she didn't.

'I don't need them,' she said, pushing away the capsules I'd given her. 'I ain't eating anything, so I don't gotta take them ones.'

'Okay,' I said. 'You don't have to. But you've got to eat

something when you can. Your body has been through a lot. You need the strength.'

'My body has been through more than you could imagine.'

I closed the door quietly; I knew Shannon wanted to tell me more, even if she was still staring at her phone.

'I've got bite marks and bruises, chunks of hair missing and chipped teef. You name it, he's done it. But I never thought he'd beat me this hard and keep on going.'

I'd read the brief police reports we had been given and knew that she was talking about her stepfather. I told her that I would need to pass on what she was telling me to the police if it might help their investigation, but that my duty of care was to look after her.

She shrugged and carried on.

'I wish he had killed me, though. I'd probably be better off.'

'I don't think so,' I said. 'You'll recover from this.'

'Yeah? And then what?' She looked at me, her blue eyes sitting in deep dark-purplish hollows, her teeth sharp and small, forehead clammy with sweat.

Shannon told me that she had run from the house after she and her stepdad had argued, and that he had chased after her and kicked and beaten her until she could barely stand. She showed me the burn marks up her arms, the freshly pink bite marks on her hands and the patches of white scalp where the pulled-out hair had never grown back after years of abuse.

'And he's seeing some ovver bird now. Mum don't even

know it; she's barely there anyway. But he still lives in our house, eating our food, shitting in our toilet.' She turned her phone around and showed me a photo from his social media page of an older man wearing a cap, his arm slung around a pouting young girl. 'She don't look old enough to even have a boyfriend, does she? She don't know what she's letting herself in for . . .'

The glow from the phone illuminated the beads of sweat on Shannon's brow. She wiped her nose with her sleeve. I wasn't sure if she was crying; her eyes were pink-rimmed and darkly shadowed from lack of sleep, lack of food and punches to the sockets.

Later, various police officers and the safeguarding team within the hospital visited Shannon. Shannon's mood was a storm: she trusted no one and her anger was as sharp as broken glass.

Alongside other nursing staff, I looked after Shannon for nearly two weeks before she was moved to a respiratory ward, deemed well enough from a cardiothoracic point of view to now have her CF taken care of before possibly being sent home. She had, however, contracted a chest infection and needed intravenous antibiotics before she could go anywhere at all.

I walked beside her wheelchair as she was taken to the respiratory ward. I spent a long time talking to the nurse who would be looking after her there. Shannon's lungs were almost healed from the attack but had been left weaker than ever; if she wasn't compliant with her CF treatment, I knew it wouldn't be long before her condition worsened. From what I heard from the safeguarding team, Shannon would be going home whilst her stepdad was awaiting trial. I wondered how she would feel travelling back from the hospital to the same place where she had been beaten to the floor, her lungs screaming out for air.

16

In London, summer arrived. The city was hot, tourists dabbled their hands in the fountains, commuters unbuttoned their shirts and tucked their ties in their pockets. In those sweltering days I thought a lot about Shannon. I imagined her walking through her estate, an ice cream van playing its wind-up chimes as it passed, a police helicopter circling overhead, the smell of fried chicken and acetone from the nail shops on the air. I imagined her looking up at the fingerprint-smeared window of her flat; how she might quicken her pace, her brow sweating, licking her lips, tasting the salt on her skin.

On my day off, I went to meet Dad at the National Gallery. I'd spent time in a café on the South Bank and walked across Westminster Bridge to get to Trafalgar Square. I stopped outside St Margaret's Church, looking in on its stained glass and medieval arches, and remembered my dad's story about when he had come here to watch his own god.

Beneath the white stone arches, Duke Ellington, the American band leader, had been rehearsing one of his Sacred Concerts with an English choir he'd not played with before. Dad was freelancing as a journalist and sitting in the front pew watching the impromptu musical meanderings.

Ellington would play a note but the choir would flatten it when they sang and they'd have to start all over again. Soon he called upon his long-term sax player, Harry Carney, to try and move things along.

Dad sat and listened.

'Harry, do your little thing here!' Ellington cried. He wanted Carney to improvise a bridge to get to the next section.

Dad told me that Carney was a great musician, a good driver and a good drinker. One afternoon back in the States, he was pulled over by the police. He had, of course, been drinking and could barely stand. The police instructed him to blow into a bag: a breathalyser test.

Carney knew how to breathe. By the time he died, he had been playing sax for fifty years, forty-five of them spent with Ellington, sucking in air and pushing it out through the gold chambers of his horn. He knew how to hold on to a note.

Dad told me that on this occasion he initiated his circular breathing technique, blowing into the bag continuously, drawing air in through his nose and simultaneously pushing air stored in his cheeks out through his mouth. The alcohol on his breath went undetected. The police were baffled – spooked – and waved him quickly on his way.

I laughed at the thought of it as I walked to meet Dad. He came up the stairs slowly, seeming to stop on every step. I asked him if he was all right, but he couldn't catch his breath. When he got to the top, he leant on the balustrade beside me and asked if we might stay a moment overlooking the square. Pigeons and tourists streaked past; a man break-danced in front of a large crowd, the bass from his speaker reverberating beneath us. From the corner of my eye I watched Dad. His shoulders heaved, his breath was ragged and clipped short, a trapped wing flapping against a cage.

Circulation

And I am aware of my heart: it opens and closes
Its bowl of red blooms out of sheer love of me.

Sylvia Plath, 'Tulips'

17

A few weeks after our trip to the National Gallery, Dad collapsed at home. He and Mum were sitting at the kitchen table eating dinner when Dad's eyes rolled to the back of his head and he slumped forward.

Mum told us that she screamed his name but he didn't respond; that she ran to catch him and became trapped between him and the kitchen table, holding up his weight with both arms and her knees.

During that long minute, our dog, Bela, padded around on the landing upstairs, the oven timer buzzed, the boiler clicked on and a squirrel leapt from the roof to the wet garden flagstones. At last Dad regained consciousness, sitting up in the chair, Mum's arms still around him, though he was unable to say what had happened. He had no recollection of the events preceding his collapse, but when he talked of the swirling moment he came round, he described a faded image of us all floating up to the surface behind his eyes. In that image, Daisy and I were children once again, the whole family huddled together in front of an old-fashioned propeller plane beneath a hot sun, our faces racked with worry.

In the summer holidays of 1997, we travelled the west coast of America. Mum and Dad took us to the Grand

Canyon, where we bundled into a small propeller plane that held six people, the black tarmac shimmering beneath us in the heat. The take-off was smooth, the sky blue and clear, but as soon as we drew close to the brown and red canyon basin, the aircraft bucked and jolted. Over the radio the pilot told us we were going to experience turbulence for a short while, but that he was doing his best to fly above the thermals that were working against the small plane.

The turbulence didn't stop. I laid my head in Mum's lap and forced sleep to come. She stroked my hair. The plane was hot and somebody had vomited. Up front, the pilot pressed a lot of buttons. Dad's eyes watched us all, moving from my sister to me and my mum running her fingers through my hair. He turned back to the front and gazed out at the sky and the rock. Below us the river widened, the canyon's edges smooth from the water that had run past it for all those years.

The great artist Leonardo da Vinci believed that the power of water running across a surface could, in time, make the entire earth 'a perfect sphere'. He was fascinated by shells and fossils preserved in rock, understanding that they owed their existence to all that had come before, rather than attributing their presence to stories of biblical floods, a more pervasive belief at the time.

Our plane shook for the whole journey. When we landed, my sister and I headed for the car, overjoyed to be away from the stubby wings and tiny wheels of the aircraft.

In the sixteenth century, Leonardo da Vinci illustrated

his findings on turbulence, sketching water flowing from above into a lower pool and the resulting curling, scrambling shape it made when the surface was disturbed. He understood the effect water could have on the earth and studied the changing flow turbulence caused, capturing the notion of waves and currents, tides and eddies with his quill and ink.

Using his knowledge of movement and grasp of flow, he questioned established thinking during the Renaissance period with regard to the role of the heart. Over a thousand years earlier, Galen, a Greek physician, had expounded his own theories on the heart and the movement of blood; most people still believed his findings, agreeing that the heart's primary role was to produce heat.

Galen wrote that the heart was the hearthstone of the body and that its central position and innate warmth was a fundamental element of life, symbolizing its deep connection to the soul. He decided that blood was divided into two distinct networks, the venous and the arterial. Venous blood was created in the liver from digested food and used as an alimentary source through the body. Meanwhile, arterial blood flowed past the lungs to the heart; it was here that he believed it acquired *pneuma* – 'breath' or 'spirit' – and, when absorbed into the bloodstream, became a vital essence providing the body with its fundamental life force. Galen believed that this blood flowed through the septum that divides the heart in two, convinced that the membrane was permeable and filled with holes, rather than through the mechanical pumping of the heart with its one-way valves.

Despite Galen's dogmatic teachings persisting, Leonardo decided to pursue his own study. He had first-hand experience of dissections, using melted wax to make a mould of the valves within a hundred-year-old man's heart after he had died. By looking at the anatomy before him, he began to question Galen's description of blood flowing back and forth through the heart via a porous membrane that separated the chambers.

Leonardo insisted that the heart was a muscle, not simply flesh, with four chambers rather than two, capable of opening and closing and thus driving blood around it. These findings differed vastly from Galen's notions that blood sloshed back and forth through two chambers. Leonardo instead wrote of eddy currents and sinewy membranes separating the chambers, helping to propel blood forward. He produced accompanying drawings to provide a mechanical account of the flow of blood that would shape the modern world's perception of the much-debated organ.

Dad went to his GP to see if she could explain why he had lost consciousness. She asked him whether he was aware he had a heart murmur, turbulence whirling beneath the stethoscope. Dad said he was, but it had never caused him any trouble.

A heart murmur can be heard by placing a stethoscope against the chest. Its occurrence is both normal and abnormal, and it is through listening to the sound of blood flowing through the heart that this classification can be distinguished. A normal murmur may be caused by increased activity and subsequent rapid blood flow: running or swimming speedy lengths. A clinician trained in listening to the intricacies of heart sounds will be able to interpret the crescendo and decrescendo, the whooshings and swishings that happen at particular times of the heart cycle, and whether the sound of turbulence – the murmur – indicates a problem requiring further investigation.

Dad was referred to the cardiologists at the local hospital, who would perform more investigations. In the meantime, blood was taken at the surgery and we were sent home.

18

In my job, I encountered blood, in some form, every day. I was familiar with its core-of-the-earth redness when aspirated straight from a well-oxygenated artery, its dull shade of bluish-red when drawn from the venous circulation. I knew the look of it when it met the air, slopping in clots to the orthopaedic surgeon's feet as he cut away muscle to get to bone during hip surgery. I had hung blood bags, primed transfusions, watched the plastic giving set change colour as the blood crept through the line, clamping it just before it reached the connector and spilt forth.

At night I'd stooped and stared down at chest drains filled nearly to the top, a litre of blood-tinged fluid bubbling like a witch's cauldron, hot and freshly emptied from a chest cavity. I'd rolled an elderly patient one morning to change the sheets beneath her and found her white thighs daubed red, sunk within deep linen vats of black blood still running out from her like an afterbirth, thick and tarry with clots from gastrointestinal bleeding. I'd mopped up sumping chest wounds with sterile gauze, attached vacuum-assisted devices to suck the ooze, held swabs to arrow-slit stab wounds until they stopped weeping, and tightened tourniquets around turgid blood vessels, breaking the skin with a small-bore needle to draw a sample.

I had become fluent in the way blood moved, smelt, how its colour could signal a patient's chances of survival.

When I first qualified as a nurse, I went to work in a central London hospital with nearly a thousand beds serving a diverse community of over seven hundred thousand people from the neighbouring boroughs. Its corridors heaved; the long passageways brought forth a steady flow of monitored beds, porters clutching the rails. Visitors bearing steaming Tupperware rode the lifts to other levels, read floor plans, leapt out of the way of yellow tube-fed children being pushed in wheelchairs and uniformed staff confidently weaving past each other, some en route to a break, others to a meeting or an emergency call.

As a newly qualified nurse, I was enlisted to the cardiac division. Over the next eighteen months, I made my way through the cardiovascular specialties, meeting people adapting to new lives without limbs on the vascular wards, keeping watch overnight on patients who had suffered heart attacks, and learning how to titrate medication for patients on the high dependency unit recovering from open-heart surgery. It was here on the HDU that I stayed, having become passionate about the life-giving, life-changing impact of cardiac surgery.

One afternoon we were preparing to receive a patient who was being stepped down to the HDU from intensive care. His chest too had whirled beneath the stethoscope, the turbulence loud in the cardiologist's ears as the patient lay unresponsive in the bed. He was now stable enough to be looked after on our unit without the need for a one-to-one nurse and a breathing machine. We had been told he had suffered an out-of-hospital cardiac arrest; his heart was still undergoing investigation to find out the cause. He was a young man with a wife and a new baby, neither of whom had yet left his side.

Farah was pushed into the HDU by two hospital porters, a senior critical-care nurse and an advanced nurse practitioner dressed in red. His bed flashed with monitors and infusions and the mobile suction machine hissed air at us as it lay at his side ready to be used. He had a tracheostomy in his throat to help him breathe and a nasogastric tube inserted to provide him with nutrition. On the monitor his heart, blood pressure, and oxygen saturations were recorded in different colours that oscillated across the screen. His observations looked stable but his big brown eyes stared blankly ahead; he didn't notice us moving around him, securing infusions to drip stands, gathering oxygen tubing from beneath the pillows to plug in at the wall. His wife waited for us to settle him on the unit, her baby cradled in her arms, a prayer mat laid across its legs.

As the weeks went on, we heard from his wife, Aisha, and his social worker that Farah had been born in Kismayo, a port city in the south of Somalia. He was just a few years older than me. His parents had sent him to the UK as a child in the hope that he could escape the fighting and start a new life with people that might be able to keep him safe here. As a young man, he had become a bus driver and navigated the city's labyrinthine streets as if he had always known them.

He and Aisha rented a flat in Stratford, overlooking the new Olympic Park. At night they would climb through the maintenance hatch at the top of the building and sit on the roof, gazing out at the stadium, the floodlights casting white sunshine over fake grass, the day lasting just that little bit longer for them up there. They looked out as far as the night would let them and Farah thought of home.

Back in Somalia the Kismayo sea wall stretched along the coast line, the port city lights glowed throughout the night. In the summer months the Indian Ocean was a hot bath, and people lay on the beach hoping to catch a breeze. Farah told his wife that as a child he would swim out and collect shells and coral from the reef and place them in the round bullet holes that were left behind in the sea-wall; holes that you'd peer through and hope to see blue sky on the other side.

One evening in Stratford, after a long shift, Farah was playing squash at the local leisure centre with some friends. He began feeling tired and had a headache so went to sit down on the benches at the side of the court. Before he could get there, he collapsed. His friends gathered frantically around him, peering down at his squirming body. He wasn't breathing. One of them knelt down and began performing cardiopulmonary resuscitation, depressing Farah's chest firmly with the heels of his palms.

The ambulance flashed its way to the front of the leisure centre and the paramedics ran in and took over. They attached Farah to the portable monitor but found no electrical activity in his heart; there wasn't a single spark they could shock back to life. They continued pumping blood around his body, using their hands intertwined on his chest, pushing down firmly. They placed a plastic tube in his mouth to protect his airway, applying oxygen to try and keep his brain alive whilst they worked on him. After fifteen minutes of CPR and administration of adrenaline, the thin trace of a heartbeat appeared on the screen, Farah's blood flow returning as if the heart muscle had finally woken up and remembered it needed to beat.

The results of his echocardiogram at the hospital revealed that he had a congenital hole in his heart: a defect in the septum, the membrane separating the chambers, which meant that blood shunted abnormally back and forth. The hole and the turbulent sloshing of blood through to the other side increased the overall volume of blood that his heart had to hold. This meant that the right side worked harder to propel blood, and thus became enlarged, stretched thin and less able to do its job effectively as a pump. The reduced blood flow caused by the poor pumping meant there were fewer minerals and electrolytes to conduct electricity in his heart, the wiring therefore faulty and at risk of short-circuiting. It also meant that he had less oxygen circulating around his body at any one time. Like a climber at altitude, his body tried to adjust to these lower levels of oxygen, which made his blood thicker and thus more prone to forming dangerous clots.

Almost two thousand years before Farah arrived at the hospital, Galen's perception of the heart was that the septum was porous and a key site of interchange. He placed great emphasis on the pores of the septum, describing permeable funnel-shaped grooves that ended almost in darkness. He believed it was through these dark pores that blood moved back and forth in order that *pneuma* be absorbed and life thus sustained.

It wasn't until William Harvey's *On the Motion of the Heart and Blood in Animals,* written in the seventeenth century, that people began to perceive the inner workings in a different way, understanding that the flow of blood was reliant on a one-way system of heart valves and contraction. For Farah, his Galenic heart meant that the blood moving back and forth through the septum had resulted in a cardiac arrest.

On the HDU, we recorded Farah's consciousness on our charts as less than half that of a person with normal functioning cognition, since his brain had been deprived of oxygen for so long during the cardiac arrest. We scored him for opening his eyes spontaneously, but he couldn't speak and he didn't move, the only flickering of life his dark eyes blinking at the room. Just a week ago he had been in his bus, driving commuters and tourists across the city; hitting a ball; cradling his new baby in his arms; gazing out at the Olympic lights. Now he lay in a hospital bed, staring up at the ceiling, the secretions from his mouth and windpipe being suctioned away by visor-wearing nurses.

Farah stayed with us on the HDU for a long time. I had recently become tracheostomy trained, and he would be the first patient with a breathing tube that I would look after. It was a night shift, handover starting at seven thirty. I had slept in the day, showered, eaten dinner and driven to work, the radio playing smooth love songs. I caught sight of my tired face in the rear-view mirror doused in brake-light red.

After handover, I went straight to see Farah. I wanted to check I had all the equipment I needed for a shift spent looking after his airway. He was producing a lot of sputum, thick, sticky secretions that needed to be cleared with suction from his throat. Inside the room was the sealed red tracheostomy bag containing all I might need in an emergency: spare tubes, saline, gauze, and tracheal dilating forceps in case the hole needed holding open if the tube came out.

I went to the storeroom and picked up more sterile gloves, suction catheter tubes, tracheostomy dressings, cleaning wipes, and inner tubes so that I could change the inside of the tracheostomy when it became encrusted with dry secretions. Then I made my way back to the side room where Farah lay, positioned on his left side with pillows to take the pressure off his bottom.

I said hello and told him my name and that I would be looking after him for the night shift. His hands were clasped around rolled-up bed linen, exercises prescribed by the physiotherapists. His thick beard had been trimmed close to his face; his wife had put oil in his hair.

She came into the room holding the baby in her arms; he had just been fed and was sleeping. Prayers played softly from the stereo on the windowsill. The whole room seemed to be drawn inwards by the centripetal repetition of the chanting, as if we were being pulled, feet gliding, towards the man lying asleep in the centre. Aisha sat beside him and lowered the side of the bed so that she could be closer. She rested a hand on his. The baby lay in her lap, milk-drunk, his mouth half open. She laid him in his pram.

'How're you?' I asked quietly.

She shrugged her shoulders, putting her head to one side. She smiled at me.

I nodded.

She removed the rolls of linen from Farah's balled fists and laid them at the end of the bed. She took the prayer mat and draped it across him instead.

In the darkness I could make out the curling Arabic calligraphy running along the edges, the outlines of petals and interlaced shapes, tessellating to make tall columns, minarets made of diamonds, scraping the star-studded sky, domes shrouding what lay beneath.

Aisha asked me when he would wake up.

I looked at Farah; his eyes were open. I nodded towards him, although I knew what she was really asking.

She stroked a strand of hair from his forehead. There was a pause and then she spoke again.

'His eyes are open through the night and the day, but when will he *wake up*?'

Farah had undergone EEG tests, an electroencephalogram to understand the electrical activity that might or might not be occurring in his brain. He was in a vegetative state, somewhere in between sleep and wakefulness. It was unclear how he would recover, and if he would wake from this in-between place. His state encompassed numerous disorders and he presented with many of them in his behaviours. He had no awareness of himself or his surroundings; his eyes roved the room without recognizing anything; both his bladder and bowel were incontinent; he gave no evidence of purposeful movement, arms lying rigid at his sides, hands in tightly locked fists, thumbs buried inside. They were not hands that held shells any more.

The doctors were not able to offer a prognosis at this early stage. His brain might recover from not receiving oxygen, but only time would tell. His heart, for the meantime, was stable. We had worked hard to restore the electrolytes in his blood to within normal ranges and his blood was being kept thin with medication so that it could pass without problem through his heart and the rest of the body. When he was well enough, the hole separating the atria would be repaired.

Aristotle believed that the heart was the seat of all intelligence and emotion, the organ most connected to a person's soul. Egyptian embalmers thought little of the brain and discarded it during mummification. The heart, however, was left intact, believed to be of use in the afterlife. In order to progress to the Field of Reeds, the heavenly realm of the ancient Egyptians, the dead person's heart would be weighed before Osiris, the Lord of the Underworld. A person who had lived a life full of good deeds would have a light heart, lighter than a feather, and would thus successfully pass the ceremony. If a heart proved too heavy, it would be thrown to the crocodile-headed Ammit, who would devour it there on the spot, its owner never allowed to transcend into the next realm.

That morning, when I got home from my night shift looking after Farah, I asked Rob to sit down at the kitchen table and take off his T-shirt. He laughed – it was cold, he said, he had only just woken up and he wanted a cup of tea – but he saw the expression on my face and obliged.

I took my stethoscope from my bag and placed the cool diaphragm on his upper chest. Rob didn't speak; just breathed deeply and let me listen. I knelt between his legs, moved the stethoscope across towards the left side of his chest, heard the full swell of his heart completing a cycle. I moved it down his ribcage, listening to the blood being pumped, straining my ears to hear the exact moment of squeeze and release.

Beneath his stone sternum I heard a carnelian sun beating a holy sequence of notes. I listened hard. I stared up at the veins in his arms, at his chest rising and falling, and at his neck, where a jugular root, plumed with valves, squirmed up to the surface to speak. The blood was loud, the heartbeat strong, regular, calling me to him.

20

During the first few weeks of my new job on the cardio-thoracic ward, just six months into being qualified as a nurse, I was invited to watch my first cardiac bypass surgery. Most new starters are encouraged to witness an open-heart procedure to better understand the patient's journey from outpatient clinic to surgery to recovery with the nurses back on the wards.

In the cool of the operating theatre I tentatively peered over the anaesthetist's shoulder to watch the surgeon's blade make a clean, almost bloodless incision down the skin of a woman's chest. I watched as the surgeon and his registrar used heat to slice through the gelatinous layer of fat beneath, finally reaching the bone, which they proceeded to cut through with a saw. The smell of brazier smoke and fireworks nights momentarily distracted me from the surgery. When I looked back, they had already flayed the chest; the bone marrow was now visible, jam-coloured and sponge-like. They worked quickly, with silver fingers, and with the chest cranked open they cut through the glistening pericardial sac to reveal the heart, the first I had ever seen.

My own heart leapt, but I tried to stay as still and quiet as possible, balancing on tiptoes on a stool by the patient's head to get a better view. The team had inserted thick garden-hose tubes in the aorta and the atrium to attach the patient to the cardiopulmonary bypass machine – the heart-lung machine. They used clamps and silk sutures to ensure they could control the flow and that the tubes would remain fixed safely in place.

It was the perfusionist, sitting nearby, whose job it was to initiate the heart-lung machine. The heart in front of me was emptied, the lungs deflated, no longer required to take breaths for themselves, since the machine would do it for them for the duration of the operation. The machine whirred to life, canisters filling up with blood, spooling it through tubes, arcing over spinning discs like a bloody rainbow bowing above a metallic sun, looping back again past pumps and filters, chrome panels, bags of fluid hooked high like Halloween piñatas waiting to be punctured. The patient could now not survive without the perfusionist's bypass machine oxygenating the body.

This machine was first successfully used on a human by John Gibbon, who developed the earliest cardiopulmonary bypass machine in 1950s Philadelphia. His skill as a doctor had been handed down from his father, grandfather, great-grandfather and great-great-grandfather before him, and he had dedicated years of study to developing ways of enhancing cardiac surgery.

That morning he operated on a young woman who had an atrial septal defect; like Farah's, a hole in the heart that allowed blood to pass back and forth abnormally through the septum. The operation took twenty-six minutes; twenty-six minutes of her life spent beating and breathing through his new machine. It worked: she recovered uneventfully and went home, her heart fixed.

When Gibbon left Jefferson University Medical Center that afternoon, he crossed the road and thought he could smell on the breeze the sweetness of bloodroot petals from the Catskill Mountains that had fallen and been carried all the way to Philadelphia by the Delaware River. He made his way home through Washington Square, the sycamore leaves green and vein-filled in the light. He walked the diagonal concrete paths of the park, his feet sore from standing, and stopped in the middle, where a fountain spurted. He closed his eyes and reflected on the operation, listening to the rush of the fountain as the water crashed to the ground and thinking back to how the heart had looked as it refilled with blood.

Back in the operating theatre in London, I watched as the senior house officer extracted a suitable vein from the patient's leg to use as a graft in the heart. Her masked face was pressed close to the flesh, peering over her glasses to check she had removed the whole vessel, cutting it away from its branches. She carefully lifted it from its bed. With one hand she held the vessel; with the other she squirted water through its lumen to clean it and check its patency. It looked like the thorny stalk of a rose without its head. She passed the vein to the scrub nurse, who placed it safely in a sterile dish whilst the surgeons continued working on the heart. The SHO bowed her head once more, clamping the branch stumps and selecting sutures to tie them off at the root, before closing the leg and wrapping it in bandages.

The surgeons took the new vessel and planted it deep within the chest, sewing it to the openings of the diseased arteries, using magnified lenses to inspect their work more closely. Blood flow was established to check the graft was working, and slowly the patient was weaned from the heart-lung machine as the operation came to an end.

The registrar inserted chest drains to remove any remaining fluid from the area, and temporary pacing wires were positioned in the outer layer of the heart to provide electrical stimulation to manage the patient's heart rate and rhythm should it not be able to conduct for itself when they awoke.

Steel wires were used to close the sternum and the chest was sutured back together. The patient was wheeled out to cardiac recovery, where they would remain breathing via a machine overnight. The nurses here would monitor vital signs closely, checking that blood pressure remained stable and the heart beat in a regular rhythm. They would use a variety of drugs to increase the strength of the heart's contractions and monitor the flow of blood, looking for early signs of bleeding. The location of the surgery, deep within the chest, meant that bleeding was often concealed, and nurses had to spot subtle signs before it was too late.

When I had more experience in cardiac nursing, I too would be able to work in cardiac recovery, but in the meantime, I would start at the beginning of the patient's journey, on the cardiothoracic ward, getting them ready for their big operation.

21

I had experience preparing a patient for theatre from my first few months as a nurse. At the start of my cardiac rotation in the central London hospital, I worked on the vascular ward, where patients were awaiting or recovering from surgery to unblock their veins and arteries; not too dissimilar from what I would come to know in cardiothoracics.

Preparing somebody for theatre means answering questions, washing and shaving the area for surgery, and removing any make-up and jewellery. Depending on the type of surgery, the patient may need to be fasted from midnight in order that they can be safely anaesthetized. Once a person is put to sleep, they are no longer in control of their airway. Fasting prior to general anaesthetic aims to reduce the volume and the acidity inside the patient's stomach, lowering the risk of them accidentally regurgitating and aspirating gastric contents into their lungs. This is a rare occurrence but a dangerous one, and through fasting, possibly allowing the patient just small sips of water beforehand, the risk is further reduced.

It was my first night shift as a qualified nurse. I was working on a busy thirty-bedded vascular ward that looked after people requiring surgery to fix the blood flow in their legs, or who had reached a point where a leg now required amputation.

I was allocated eight patients, some recently admitted, some post-operative and recovering and one awaiting surgery the next day. There were three nurses on the shift, including myself. We took our handovers from the day staff and went to meet our patients. The nurse in charge for the night was called Matilda. She had been working predominantly night shifts for the last twenty years. We hadn't worked together before, and she draped her arm softly around my shoulders as she discussed my patients with me, then slipped a Chinese takeaway menu across the desk and tapped one of the dishes. She looked me in the eye and smiled; she had one gold tooth that gleamed in the light.

'Special soup,' she said. 'It will get us through the night.'

I nodded and took the menu; it was creased as if it had been folded and unfolded hundreds of times on night shifts gone by. I looked back and saw Matilda greeting her own patients for the night with jazz hands. She didn't look like someone who lived on a diet of Chinese take-away and night shifts.

I walked slowly down the corridor, my mind full of what I had to do. What time should I start my drug round? What time should I start mixing my intravenous medica-tion? What time should I start recording observations on my patients: blood pressure, respiration rate, and neuro-vascular observations on the post-operative patient to make sure their limbs were still warm and blood-filled after the surgery? I could already hear buzzers ringing at the other end of the ward, the linoleum lit up by the flashing orange call bells.

I spent my first night shift as a student nurse on a quiet orthopaedic ward in the hospital up the hill where I had had my own surgery as a teenager and where Daisy worked in the birth centre. The ward overlooked the park next to the hospital and beside the school I had gone to. I could hear the green parakeets settling in their nests for the night. After that, the only sound came from the squeak and creak of arms and legs held in pulleys and traction to keep their broken bones straight overnight.

I was given the second break, and the nurse in charge told me to take it in the staff room. To my surprise, she had set up a camp bed in the middle of the room, with the sheets perfectly turned down over a hospital blanket. It looked like a mirage after seven hours on my feet and midnight already a couple of hours gone. Despite this, I remember not feeling tired. I had been so nervous about my first night shift that my brain felt wired, buzzing and alert, ready to learn. Nevertheless, I got into the bed.

There was a knock at the door; it was the nurse in charge. I quickly kicked off the sheets, thinking perhaps the bed wasn't actually meant for me. She smiled and ushered me back into it. She advised me not to set my phone alarm as I was right next to the female patients' bay and it might disturb them. She assured me she would wake me up in an hour's time, and closed the door softly behind her. I lay there in the dark, listening to the sounds of the hospital around me. Distant lifts being called, felt-lined doors closing, doctors' bleeps, and soft-soled shoes on shiny floors . . .

It turned out to be the longest one-hour break I had ever experienced. When the knock on the staff room door eventually came, I rolled over quickly and checked my phone: it was six o'clock in the morning! I had been asleep for four hours!

I jumped out of the camp bed, my student uniform creased, my hair down and shoes kicked off in the corner of the room. When I opened the door, I saw the smiling faces of my qualified colleagues, all three of them barely able to contain their laughter.

'Did you sleep well?' the nurse in charge whispered, trying her best to hide her grin.

'I am so sorry,' I said. 'I slept through my alarm.'

She nodded. 'No you didn't, remember?'

I thought back to the early hours and remembered being advised not to set it. I looked at her and her face broke into a smirk. The other nurses laughed and one of them pulled me close and hugged me.

'It's okay,' she said. 'Don't look so worried. You have another forty years of night shifts; we thought we'd start you off gently.' I could hear her heartbeat through her uniform.

'But you three didn't get to take your breaks,' I said.

The nurse who was hugging me waved her hand.

'We rested,' she said. 'And we talked. It was a quiet shift.'

'Come on.' The nurse in charge turned back to the ward. 'Mr Martin's wound has been oozing all night, and it's your turn to dress it.'

I straightened my uniform, tied my hair back and grabbed my shoes. The morning sun was peeping through the windows and the ward was waking up.

Back on my first night shift as a qualified nurse on the vascular ward, I felt the weight of my responsibilities upon me. I was no longer a student. These were my patients for the night. They relied on me, and the safe keeping of their hearts, lungs and limbs depended on my skill as a nurse.

Matilda was working in the middle of the ward; I could hear her pushing the drug trolley into the bay. The vascular ward was located in the basement; even when morning came, there would be no natural light. The windows opened out to brick walls and concrete, as if we were in the depths of an underground bunker. I had read that night shifts are made more bearable if you can expose yourself to light overnight. The body has an internal twenty-four-hour clock that dictates when to sleep and when to wake, known as the circadian rhythm. The part of the brain that controls this rhythm can be tricked by exposure to bright light into thinking that it's daytime, which in turn makes you more alert. Night shifts shrouded in darkness are harder to bear, punctuated by heavy-lidded eyes and yawning mouths.

'Nurse!' I heard somebody call from the quiet of a bay.

I turned to see who needed me. A little old lady had spilt her tea on the sheets.

'I'm sorry, love.' She looked up at me, her hands raised in apology. I checked to see if she had hurt herself, but the tea was so cold it had grown a skin, and once she was tucked back in with clean sheets and a blanket, she was asleep before I could ask her if she needed anything else.

I made my way to the side rooms. The post-operative patient I was keen to see was having a scan, and so I went to check on the patient awaiting theatre tomorrow.

Louis was a seventy-year-old man due to have vascular surgery on his right leg. He had been experiencing increasing pain when walking short distances. He was booked in for a femoral popliteal bypass, which would divert his blood circulation away from the blocked vessel no longer providing adequate blood flow to his leg muscle. This blockage meant that his calf was starved of oxygen-rich blood and was having to cope without, much like a runner who develops cramp mid-race, stopping and clutching their leg, waiting for the circulation to replenish the limb and the pain to subsequently diminish.

I introduced myself and took his observations, recording them on the computer. I told him that I would help to prepare him for surgery the next day; that I would need to shave the hair on his body and he would have to wash with antiseptic scrub. Louis seemed relaxed about the operation; he continued unpacking his suitcase, neatly folding his pyjamas and placing them in the bedside cabinet as I spoke to him. He smiled at me when I asked if he felt nervous, and shook his head.

'I'll be pleased to have it done,' he said. 'Then I can get on with my life. This leg has caused me pain for such a long time.' He tapped his right leg beneath his trousers.

Louis' condition was not uncommon for his age and

lifestyle. He had recently given up smoking and changed his diet, but his cholesterol had been high for many years, and that and the cigarettes, as well as a history of heart disease in his family, had contributed to the layer of fatty deposits that had now built up inside his arteries.

These fatty deposits are called atheroma, derived from the Greek word *athere*, meaning 'groats' or 'gruel', since the consistency is thick and porridge-like when scraped away from the vessel. They are the same type of plaques found by the archaeologists at the British Museum who put Egyptian mummies through the CT scanner, revealing their furred-up arteries and offering insight into their diet and lifestyle thousands of years ago.

Louis swam every morning and was keen to have the operation done with so that he could go back to his routine. He would be competing in an over-65s fund-raising event in a couple of months' time at the local leisure centre and had already had numerous people donate money to the cause. He was eager to race.

In the weeks before his operation, he had attended a pre-assessment clinic, where the surgeon had reminded him that he might not be up to the swim, but the event was motivating him to get through the surgery and prepare himself for his recovery afterwards. He told me he would be staying with his partner, who had taken some time off work in order to look after him at home.

'She's good to me,' he grinned. 'I'm twenty years older than her and I'm sure she'd much rather be at work instead of nursing me, but what can I say? I'm a lucky man.'

'I'm sure you both look after each other,' I said.

He smiled and nodded. 'I didn't think I'd find someone at my age . . .'

He zipped his toiletry bag and placed it on his neatly folded clothes, then turned to face me, sitting on the edge of his bed.

'So,' he said. 'You need me washed, shaved and shined, is that right?'

'That's right,' I said. 'I'll see to a few other patients first and come back to you with everything I need, if that's okay?'

'Right you are!' He swung his legs up onto the bed and took his book from the cabinet. 'See you soon!' He flicked on his bedside light.

By the time I had finished the rest of my tasks, it was almost midnight. I felt behind in my work and knew it was unfair to leave Louis' preparation so late, but numerous patients were bedbound and had required assistance using the bedpan, and the medication round was delayed as I needed routine tablets to be prescribed by the doctor on call. When I came to look at the prescription charts, I realized I had more intravenous antibiotics to administer than I'd thought, and one patient was complaining of chest pain so I stopped everything to run ECGs and take blood. At eleven in the evening my post-operative patient had come back from her scan, and I called the doctor as her foot no longer felt as warm as it had. A junior doctor was taking care of all the surgical wards overnight and had a collection of bleeps attached to his belt like a gunslinger.

'You called?' he said. He wasn't annoyed but I could see

he was already looking at his other bleep and a call he had not yet responded to.

'Mrs Shorter's foot feels cooler than it did before.'

'Obs?' he asked, checking that she was stable.

'All fine,' I replied. She wasn't scoring on our early-warning trigger chart; it was just that the foot no longer felt warm.

'Doppler?' he said. The Doppler is a small ultrasound device used to listen for blood flow.

I shook my head.

He took the Doppler out of the drawer and went to Mrs Shorter's room. I followed, but soon another buzzer went and I tended to that patient instead. By the time I had sorted out a malfunctioning intravenous drip, the doctor had finished and was cleaning the Doppler probe with a wipe.

'All fine,' he said. One of his bleeps went off. 'Good flow. Keep doing obs.'

I nodded and he was gone.

Eventually I went back to Louis. He was in the same position I had left him. When he saw me, he smiled and slipped a bookmark into his book. I apologized to him but he wouldn't hear of it.

'Not an issue,' he said. 'Now, what's first?'

'Let's do the theatre checklist,' I said, sitting down beside the bed.

'Great! This is where you ask about wooden legs and shrapnel, right?'

'Almost,' I said.

Most of the questions I could tick without even

checking with Louis; they related to whether I had appropriately attached named wristbands and whether he was wearing compression stockings. When I reached the end of the list, I asked him whether he had any false or loose teeth.

'A plate at the top,' he said, showing me with his finger.

'That's fine,' I said. 'We'll put it somewhere safe in the morning. Latex allergy?'

'No,' he said.

'Do you have a pacemaker?'

He shook his head.

'Any prosthetics?'

'Nope,' he said. 'Just the wooden leg, like I said.' He raised an eyebrow at me.

'Any metalwork at all in your body, hips, knees, joints?'

He shook his head again, and then stopped. 'Jewellery count?'

I glanced up. 'You can take that off in the morning,' I told him, looking for a ring on his finger.

'Body piercings,' he said. 'I have some body piercings.' He pulled up his T-shirt to show me a large nipple ring.

'That will have to come out,' I said, and looked back at the checklist.

'And one here as well.' He indicated towards his groin.

'Ah . . .' I said. 'Will you be able to remove that? Perhaps when you have your shower, you could try and take both of them out?'

He grimaced and laughed a little.

'They're both new. I haven't taken them out since I had them done.'

I completed the checklist and left Louis to shower and try and take out his piercings. I would shave him afterwards to keep the area clean and accessible for the surgeons, and then he would shower once more in the morning.

It was midnight and most of the patients seemed to be sleeping. I wandered back to the nurses' station, where Matilda was sitting.

'There you are!' she said. Maribel, the bank nurse, was parking her drug trolley and folding her handover sheet back into her pocket. Her pen torch was still glowing inside her uniform.

'I'm not quite finished.' I leant on the desk. 'I'm still getting my man prepared for theatre.'

'Do you need help?' Matilda said.

I shook my head.

'I think we missed our slot for special soup.' She sat back in the chair and stretched. 'Let's decide breaks. Does anybody have a problem with me taking first break, then I'll be back out nice and early to help with any leftover tasks and be on the floor for the rest of the shift.'

Neither of us minded.

'If you need me for anything, just come in,' she said; she'd already untied her laces to rest her feet.

I went to check on Louis. He was finished with his shower and back in his room with his hospital gown on.

'How did it go?' I asked.

'I got one,' he said, gesturing to his chest. 'I'm really sorry, I just can't unscrew the other one. I assume it will have to come out?'

'It will,' I said.

I shut the door to his room and shaved the hair from his legs and groin, making sure the skin I didn't need exposed was covered.

'Right,' I said. 'Let me get some gloves . . .' I took a pair of gloves from the wall and attempted to remove the piercing from Louis' penis. It held fast; the ball bearing wouldn't move.

'I'm so sorry,' Louis said.

'It's okay,' I said. 'I'm sorry if I'm hurting you.' I held the metal between my fingers and tried to twist, but it wouldn't move. 'Perhaps you could try again?'

I left Louis in the privacy of his room to have another go at removing the piercing. Maribel was sitting at the nurses' station computer, writing up her notes.

'I've got a problem,' I said quietly to her.

She looked up. 'Are you okay?' she said. I had seen Maribel before when I took over on the day shift. She was an experienced nurse who had worked for fifteen years in her home country of the Philippines and another five years in Saudi Arabia before moving to the UK.

'Everything's fine,' I said. 'But the man I'm preparing for theatre has some . . . metalwork.'

She frowned. 'Hip?' she said. 'That's okay.'

'Penis,' I said. 'I can't get it out.'

'Oh,' she said. She looked up to the side as if sifting through her wealth of experience to provide an answer for me. 'Would you like me to try?'

I nodded.

Maribel went to Louis' room and returned soon after.

'It's stuck,' she said. 'You will have to ring the doctor and tell him.'

I thought of the junior doctor with the bleep belt.

I bleeped him, but there was no response. I was sure he was in the middle of another busy night-shift call.

'Try the registrar,' Maribel said.

She must have noticed my expression.

'It's okay, Ms Madeira is a kitten. I don't know why everybody is scared of her.'

'I've seen her on ward rounds,' I said. 'She gets so cross. She shouts all the time; even the patients are frightened of her.'

Maribel laughed.

'His surgery will be cancelled if you don't get that padlock out.'

'Oh, don't . . .' I said. I stared down at the paperwork I had prepared: the theatre checklist, the blood results, CT report, ECGs, all the information that had been assembled to get Louis this far.

'I don't know.' Maribel turned back to the computer. 'Why would you want to lock your penis together anyway?' She tutted and continued to type.

I looked at the clock. Matilda still had forty minutes left of her break. I didn't want to disturb her.

I picked up the phone and bleeped the registrar on call. She was senior, months away from a consultancy post at another London hospital. She would be wondering why I was bleeping her when there was a perfectly good doctor on call covering the wards. But he hadn't responded and I had seen how busy he was. The thought of Louis' operation being cancelled over this made my stomach sink.

Five minutes passed, and then the phone rang, cutting through the quiet. Maribel nudged me as if I hadn't heard it.

'Hello, Ward Sixteen, Staff Nurse speaking.'

'I had a bleep.' It was Ms Madeira; her voice sounded far away.

'I'm so sorry to disturb you . . .' I began.

'What is it?'

'Mr Sinclair. He's having a fem-pop bypass tomorrow.'

'I know that.'

'He has a genital piercing I can't remove.'

There was silence down the line. I tried to imagine what the senior registrar was doing.

'A genital piercing?'

'Yes,' I said.

'And you can't remove it?'

'No,' I said. 'I've tried, we all have.'

'It has to be removed before surgery.'

'Yes,' I said.

'Get Karl,' Ms Madeira ordered.

'I think he's on another ward, I can't get through,' I said quietly.

There was silence again. I thought I could hear the hum of a vending machine in the background. I imagined Ms Madeira's face lit up in white-blue.

'You want me to attend?'

'I'm so sorry,' I said.

'I can't believe this . . .' She hung up and I heard the dial tone.

Maribel looked at me.

'Well?' she said. 'Is she coming?'

'I think so,' I replied. 'Can't be sure.'

I sat and waited at the desk. Forty minutes passed slowly. Matilda came up the corridor carrying a flask of steaming coffee, a cardigan wrapped around her.

'All okay?' she said, and yawned.

'Ms Madeira is coming,' Maribel said.

Matilda looked from Maribel's face to mine.

'Ms Madeira? Why, what happened? Is somebody sick? Who is it?' Her eyes scanned the patients' name board.

'No . . . nobody.' I took out my handover sheet and twisted it between my fingers. 'The man I'm preparing for theatre, it's just . . . I can't remove his penis piercing.'

Matilda clamped her hand over her mouth.

'Eh!' she squealed. 'And you called Ms Madeira for that?' She held her laugh quivering between her lips.

'Don't!' I said. 'I'm so scared!'

'Oh my goodness,' she said, but she was smiling at me, her head tilted to one side as if trying to understand my decision-making.

'I told her to call . . . Other doc not responding,' Maribel said, crunching on the crisps she'd brought.

'Maybe I'll make myself busy for her arrival.' Matilda looked around the ward as if pretending to find somewhere to hide.

We all tried not to laugh.

'Go and wait for her,' Matilda said, and pretended to

slap my bottom to move me out of the chair. 'Good luck,' she said. 'You'll need it.'

Ms Madeira arrived an hour after I had rung her. I had gone to the storeroom to see if there was anything I could have prepared for her arrival, but I couldn't find anything. She was wearing a black suit with a thick gold necklace peeping above her collar and a handbag with a chunky gold clasp strapped across her chest.

'Hello, Doctor,' I said. I was thankful there were no buzzers ringing, but I felt reassured that Matilda and Maribel would tend to them whilst they knew I was busy with the registrar.

'Where is he?' she said.

I hadn't had any contact with Ms Madeira before but had seen her on the day shifts. When she led the ward round, people only spoke when they were invited to, and if a scan hadn't been ordered or a blood test not yet received, she would shout at whomever she believed to be the culprit. She was known to lose her temper in front of patients, and nurses would often have to reassure them afterwards that she was much more relaxed in theatre.

I showed her into Louis' room. He was asleep. She turned the lights on and he woke.

'Mr Sinclair,' she greeted him. 'Your surgery is tomorrow. Can I look at this?' She signalled towards his lower half and he removed the blanket and his underwear quickly.

I covered as much of him as I could so that only the required part was exposed.

Ms Madeira dropped to her knees. I went to raise the bed so that she wouldn't have to kneel, but as I did, she shot me a look, and so I stopped and she remained there on the floor.

I knelt on the other side of the bed, ready to assist.

'Okay?' I half smiled at Louis. He nodded and rested his head back with his eyes closed. He said *sorry* very quietly once again.

'Hold,' Ms Madeira said to me. I held Louis' penis between two gloved fingers.

The doctor examined the piercing, assessing where she would begin. As she tried to unscrew the ball bearing, I held the penis as still and upright as I could, but I could feel my fingers slipping in the clamminess of my glove.

Louis had his arms behind his head with his eyes closed. This must have been mortifying for him.

After a few seconds, I chanced a look at Ms Madeira's face. Her dark eyes were focused on her fingers working quickly beneath the strip lights as if she were a burglar trying to pick a lock. I could see why she might have chosen to specialize in vascular surgery: her fingers were long and slim, almost as if they were surgical instruments themselves. It seemed as if she had a strategy, but every time I thought the ball had unscrewed, she would bite her lip and sigh, indicating that it had not.

'Any luck?' Louis ventured.

'Not yet, Mr Sinclair,' Ms Madeira said.

Outside the door, the ward was quiet. I hoped neither Matilda nor Maribel would peer through the glass. It would certainly be a sight to tell the day staff about in the morning: the two of us hunched over Louis' groin, fingers intertwined as if performing witchcraft together.

The doctor continued. I had never kept still for so long; I could feel my thighs shuddering and my hand starting to cramp, but I wouldn't let go.

'*Graças a Deus!*' Ms Madeira said suddenly. 'It's moving.'

Louis wiped his brow. I felt my hand relax a little.

'We've done it.' She pulled the piercing free.

I glanced at her and saw she was looking at me. I nodded.

'You have a good steady hand,' she said, and with that she stood up, removed her gloves, straightened her trousers, washed her hands and bid us both goodnight.

Louis and I smiled at each other. We both said sorry at the same time and then agreed not to say it again.

'Please get some sleep now,' I said.

He nodded and tucked himself in.

'See you in the morning,' I added.

'*Graças a Deus!*' he replied as I closed the door behind me.

22

After the vascular ward, I continued on my cardiac rotation around the hospital wards to understand the different specialties within the division. A year into the rotation, I was settled on the cardiothoracic ward.

Before a run of night shifts, I stayed at my parents' house in the daytime, sleeping soundly, away from the busy road and noisy upstairs neighbours of my own flat. In the half-light of the evening, Dad and I watched the news, sitting in the reclining chairs in the living room. It had been a few months since he had collapsed at the kitchen table. The rain tapped the skylights, clicking against the glass like planets knocking their rings together. The TV streaked blue and white against the walls. Dad had his slippered feet up on the footrest.

I was tired after sleeping through the day. I sipped hot coffee and thought about the shift ahead, the cold walk down the hill to the station, the wet-windowed train, the lights of the hospital blinking above the railway bridge, a great ship navigating through the dark.

I looked over at Dad, the little white mint he was sucking poking out from the side of his mouth. I watched him, waiting for him to pull it back in. He didn't. The mint hung from his lip, a chalky pebble waiting to topple.

'Dad?' I said.

He didn't look at me; his eyes were fixed on the TV.

I said it again. This time I stood in front of the screen. He looked up as if seeing me for the first time.

'Are you okay?' I asked, though I could see he was not.

When he opened his mouth to speak, he licked the mint away. His lips formed around the beginning of a word that couldn't be spoken.

'Dad?' I said. 'What's wrong?'

He looked cross. I'd not seen that expression before. In the darkness of the room, he appeared young again, his face set in a way he might have arranged it when his mum reprimanded him for staying out too late, or for leaving gun grease on the kitchen table before dinner.

'Talk to me, Dad.'

He tried to speak, but broken sounds fell through splintered gaps. He waved his hands as if trying to catch them before they hit the floor.

The rain was louder now against the skylights.

Dad wound his hands in circles, slowly at first, then faster as the words tumbled further from his grasp. He blew out air; the sentences just wouldn't finish any more.

'I . . .' he said. 'I . . . want . . . It's . . .'

'Dad?' I said. 'I think you're having a stroke.' I examined his face. 'Dad,' I repeated. 'Smile at me.'

He couldn't; he frowned and tried to speak again instead. He looked exhausted with the effort. I took his arms in mine, raised them up and let them fall. He was able to control them well; they landed back at his sides smoothly, without dropping.

'Talk to me again, Dad,' I said, but it was the same: the words were cracked and lay like rubble at our feet.

'We're going to have to go to hospital,' I said. 'But everything's going to be okay, you're going to be fine.' My heart was beating fast.

Dad shook his head, but I helped him get up, slip his arms into his coat and put on a hat. I could feel the rain whooshing beneath the door. He kept his slippers on and we hurried to the car.

At A&E, I told the receptionist that I thought Dad was having a stroke. I told them that he had rated positive on the stroke assessment tool and therefore time was vital in reversing any effects of the blocked blood flow.

The receptionist nodded; she had seen this before. I was grateful.

We sat down and were quickly called in to be triaged. The nurse took Dad's blood pressure, which was too high. His pulse was slow, regular but slow. We were called into A&E majors and Dad lay down on the trolley. He rested his eyes but I wouldn't let him sleep. His words were more formed now, as if the cracks had been glued and pressed together for a time. I'd called Mum. She was on her way.

The doctor came in. I watched in silence as he performed a physical examination. He raised Dad's arms and made him stick out his tongue. He touched his own nose and made Dad copy his actions. Dad did this well.

My heart felt as if it was barely beating. Time was slow. I held Dad's wet hat in my hands, stroked the herringbone stripes as if trying to read his palm lines from my place on the chair. I ran my fingers across the fabric to see what the night would hold for us.

Dad took off his shoes and socks, removed his coat and allowed the doctor to feel his calves and listen to his heart with a stethoscope. I thought of the murmur, the turbulence, Dad's slow heartbeat and the silver plane jolting hot and white above the canyon like an electric shock.

He tried to speak, but couldn't.

'It's okay,' the doctor said. 'We'll get you sorted. I'm going to get my senior to assess you.'

Dad was wheeled to Resus. Here he was hooked up to the cardiac monitor and a blood pressure cuff was applied. He lay back once more, eyes closed, chest exposed, bare and open to the ceiling, arms splayed at his sides with blood being drawn.

I wanted to call out to him, but the nurses surrounded him.

The consultant soon arrived. As she did, Dad suddenly became able to speak again, the words flowing forth like a clear stream breaking through a tangle of sticks and leaves. The sound of his voice as he greeted her was smooth and familiar, filling every space I knew. The hour without it had been silent, anechoic, deep and black. In the car, it had been so quiet, it had felt as if we were spinning silently through space, dark and empty and soundless like the moment just before the earth exploded into existence.

I sat there and listened to the richness of that voice that had called to me upstairs, school-morning landing calls;

chocolate cereal, holding hands, tobacco-stained fingers, wet ferns, walking to school in the rain.

'I think you've suffered a TIA,' the consultant said. 'A temporary blockage of blood supply to your brain caused by a clot getting in the way.'

Dad nodded.

'The clot has most likely passed now and that is why you're starting to get better.'

'Can I go home then, Doc?' he grinned.

'I want to keep you in,' she said. 'Just for tonight, to monitor your heart and your brain.'

'Yes, Dad, you must stay,' I said. I took his hands and held them tightly in my own. I felt the backs of them, piebald hands of pink and white, hands that had scooped me up from the river, hands that were now warm and tucked in mine.

When Dad was discharged home, he received a letter inviting him to attend the cardiology department, where they would run tests on his heart to find out why he had fainted at the table, and had the mini stroke. He wore a tape that recorded his heart's electrical activity over a day and a night, three sticky probes attached to his chest and a box tucked in his pocket. After that, he underwent an echocardiogram at the hospital to look at the physical structures of his heart.

Heart conditions fall into two main categories: a problem with the electricity or a problem with the plumbing. Dad's rested with the latter. A few days later, we received a letter in the post from the cardiothoracic department at the hospital I worked at in central London. The test had revealed that Dad would need to be seen urgently by the team. They had given him a diagnosis of severe aortic stenosis: one of the valves in his heart had become so narrowed that blood was struggling to pass. It was the cause of his loss of consciousness at the kitchen table, his shortness of breath, his mini stroke and the turbulence whirling in his chest.

23

Back at the hospital I worked in, Anna's heart valves needed fixing too. As a child in the north-east of Poland, a throat infection had left her knees and ankles sore to walk on. Through the illness she had lain beneath the sheets feverish and fatigued, her mother bringing her raspberry syrup tea and dabbing her face with a damp cloth as she fought away vivid dreams.

Anna had moved to the UK in her twenties, securing a job as a hostess in a hotel and restaurant in Mayfair, greeting and seating diners when they arrived. She had first lived in west London with three other people from eastern Europe: two men who worked in the kitchen and a young woman who cleaned the endless crushed-velvet rooms of the hotel.

Anna stayed in this job for twenty-five years, working her way up until she found herself managing a chain of six high-end hotel restaurants across the city. She owned her own flat in Kensington above a flower shop, and in springtime fell asleep breathing in the smell of delphiniums and cut daffodils from the shop floor.

Now sixty years old, she had come to the cardiac clinic in London complaining of feeling short of breath, thinking nothing of the childhood sore throat, the days spent at church afterwards, wrapped up warm, thanking God for giving her her voice back after she had been struck down with illness.

The echocardiogram revealed that two of her valves were scarred from the rheumatic fever she had contracted as a child. The hinges of her heart were now stiff and no longer opening properly to let the blood through.

Anna was listed for cardiothoracic surgery; she would have the two valves replaced and spend time recovering with us on the high dependency unit, and later on the ward when she was getting ready to be discharged.

Anna was a small, slim woman; you could see the muscles moving beneath her skin like ripples. She looked twenty years younger than she was, her white-blonde hair cut into a bob so that you could see the porcelain curve of her neck. Most days she wore a woolly hat with a bobble, and a pink nightie from the linen cupboard. She was quiet, never complained, and had an open-eyed expression like a nocturnal animal.

Her surgery was uneventful, the valves replaced with mechanical ones because she was relatively young and the doctors wanted them to last for the rest of her life. Since they were metallic rather than tissue, Anna would need to have her blood kept thin using medication for as long as she lived. This would take some time to get used to, some readjusting of the dose, but most patients with mechanical heart valves were successfully anticoagulated and followed up in the community. The flow of blood through the strong metal leaflets of her new valves created an audible clicking noise. When she lay back to rest on the hospital bed, her new heart cogs would tick, amplified by her sleep-drawn mouth, marking the passage of time in the hospital air.

Anna had been brought up from Cardiac Recovery the day after her surgery. She needed few infusions to keep her supported as she was recovering well, and the day after arriving with us, she was up and walking around her bed space, free from intravenous drips and monitoring devices.

As with most cardiothoracic patients leaving theatre, the surgeons had inserted temporary pacing wires in her chest, sitting in the outer layer of her heart and threaded through so that they lay above her skin. Beneath her gown the two blue wires trailed loosely down her stomach, each ending in a thin silver needle plugged into a pacing box, which was brick-like, with dials and buttons and flashing LEDs. The box stayed connected to her at all times and had extra batteries nearby in case it ran low. Since the operation, Anna had become dependent on the external pacemaker to keep her heart beating; her own internal rhythm had not yet restored itself.

When the doctors came round each morning to review her heart, they fiddled with the dials on the pacing box to see whether her own rhythm would kick in. It never did. Either the heart muscle was still too swollen from surgery to conduct electricity properly, or it had become damaged during the operation, meaning the circuit had become permanently disrupted. Since it was impossible to tell which, the team decided to wait and watch. Perhaps the swelling would subside and her normal electrics would reboot the system, allowing us to remove the external pacing box.

Days passed. Anna wandered back and forth to the toilet with the pacing box, but soon the team restricted her from doing this, worried that it might become detached and Anna would collapse somewhere far from emergency equipment. It was too risky. She would now have to use a commode placed by the side of her bed, brought to her by a nurse or a healthcare assistant when she pressed her call bell.

Over the next couple of days, friends from her church visited, but Anna drifted off to sleep during their conversations; she had been awake in the night having blood drawn, the alarms on the monitors not letting her fall back to sleep afterwards.

Early the following week, the doctors tested her heart once more. They turned the external pacing box off and watched what happened. Anna put one hand out as if trying to see in the dark, shaking her head and calling for the box to be switched on again. The screen showed her heartbeat dropping from its artificially driven sixty beats per minute to fifty, forty, thirty and twenty-five, so low that it was making her feel dizzy and nauseous. Any lower and it might stop beating completely. The doctors cranked the dial and her heartbeat returned to a regular sixty beats per minute, controlled by the silver needles conducting electricity in her heart wall.

That afternoon, the electrophysiologists came to see Anna. They talked to her about the electricity in her heart, explaining that it was conducted by a pathway of specialized cells. Generated in the sinoatrial node – which they described to her as the heart's natural pacemaker – the conducting cells transmitted an electrical impulse causing a contraction, pushing blood out from the atrium, through the valves and into the ventricles below. From here the spark travelled to the atrioventricular node, where it slowed for a moment, allowing the heart to refill with blood.

They told her it was here that her problem lay. They described how the communication between top and bottom of the heart had been disturbed by the surgery and so they no longer worked together. In a normal functioning heart, the pathway would continue down the bundle of His, through the bundle branches to the Purkinje fibres, where it could complete a full electrical circuit, a perfect heartbeat that kept blood perfusing the rest of the body.

By the next morning, it was confirmed. Anna's heart rhythm would not recover. The electrics of her heart had been damaged during the valve surgery and she was now in complete heart block. She would require a permanent pacemaker.

Whilst electrical malfunction after cardiac surgery is common, the dysfunction can be an overriding cause of morbidity unless intervention is planned. Despite this, patients often come out of major cardiac surgery, go on to require a permanent device and can still be home and recovering well within the week. The pacemaker operation does not take long: a small pocket is made in the upper left of a person's chest and the lighter-sized device tucked in, voltage calibrated and the patient neatly sewn back up.

Anna was listed for a pacemaker the next day in the catheterization laboratory, but when her latest blood test result came back, it revealed her inflammatory markers were raised, meaning that an infection might be brewing. This was not unexpected: she had been a patient in the hospital for many weeks now, the silver conducting wires still nestled in the wall of her heart like alien antennae. The cardiac team cancelled her pacemaker procedure, deeming it unsafe to operate on a person with a suspected infection.

We helped Anna into bed; she was exhausted. The doctors wanted another blood test in the morning to see whether she might be able to have the pacemaker the next day. We had all become familiar with her pink-nightie presence on the unit, the bobble hat pulled over her eyes as she tried to drift off to sleep. That evening she lay in bed rubbing oil onto her hands that her church friends had brought in for her. Soon the whole unit smelt of sandalwood and ginger.

Just as the lights had been dimmed, sleeping tablets dispensed, pillows rearranged, Anna called out: a seam-splitting cry that ripped across the starless night. The black windows looked elongated in the darkness, tall and empty of light, as she pulled at her nightdress in the dark corner of the room.

The nurses ran to her. She was panting for breath, ripping at the nightie, clawing it from her chest as if the fabric were crushing stones placed upon her to press her into the ground.

'It's okay,' one of the nurses said. 'Try to relax.' She attempted to place Anna's legs back in bed, the wires of her temporary pacing box wrapped precariously around them.

'Are you feeling sick?' another asked.

'What's going on?' A patient's drowsy voice drifted out from the darkness. One of the nurses rushed to the end of the unit to draw the curtains around the other sleeping patients.

Anna was quick and combative. In an instant she had leapt from the bed and thrown herself to her knees on the floor, arms outstretched against the shiny linoleum. The sticky electrodes had peeled from her chest, the cardiac monitor no longer able to pick up a trace.

The nurses looked up at it frantically.

The pacing box clattered down beside her but remained attached. Anna's heart was still beating but the nurses were unable to see the rhythm or rate on the screen.

Somebody bleeped the on-call doctor.

They drew the curtains around Anna and desperately tried to put her back in bed. She was gasping for breath, waving her arms in front of her as if falling from a height and bracing for impact.

'I'm going to die!' she shouted loudly into the night. 'I'm going to die here.'

'Shh.' The nurses tried to calm her. 'Anna, let's get you into bed, get you some painkillers, check your blood pressure. Can you tell us what's wrong?'

One of them managed to attach the blood pressure cuff to Anna's arm. She pressed the auto-inflate button; the cuff inflated and quickly deflated with a hiss like a balloon expending its air.

Anna's blood pressure wouldn't read.

The registrar and the SHO arrived within minutes.

Anna was reattached to the cardiac monitor, the pacing box was given to the SHO and everybody stepped back, waiting to read the trace of her heart.

The intravenous cannula had been pulled out of her skin and now dripped wetly into the bed sheets beside her. One of the nurses quickly turned it off and got rid of the sharp.

The monitor came to life above Anna's head, the green lines of her heart's trace revealing a rapid rate over one hundred and sixty beats per minute.

The nurse tried to get another blood pressure reading, but again the cuff deflated, hissing into thin air before recording anything. She ran from behind the curtain to fetch another piece of equipment. They needed a blood pressure reading. A nurse from the ward put out the cardiac arrest call. This would alert the resuscitation team that there was an imminent cardiac arrest on the HDU and full support from the hospital crash team was needed.

The registrar ordered the chest-opening trolley so that he could reopen the sternal incision they had made in surgery just over a week before. He needed to cut through the metal wires, retracting the bones in order to re-expose the heart and identify what the problem was.

A nurse shouted for the emergency drugs.

It was too dark on the unit. The healthcare assistant turned on all the lights and reassured the sleepy patients. Anna was still thrashing about beneath the sheets, though she no longer had enough breath to speak or scream.

A nurse had applied a non-rebreather oxygen mask and Anna pulled at it constantly.

The registrar ripped the sterile gown and gloves from the trolley; a nurse tied the gown for him and arranged the equipment he would need to cut open Anna's chest there and then in the corner of the unit beneath the strip lights.

All of a sudden, Anna roared, a scream like a person possessed, as if held captive inside her own body. One of the nurses tried to settle her, stroking her, pleading with her to try and relax whilst the doctor prepared to put her to sleep.

A cardiologist arrived and performed an urgent echocardiogram. It revealed the source of the problem immediately: a cardiac tamponade, an excessive accumulation of blood inside the envelope that carries the heart, hindering its ability to beat since it is so weighed down with its own blood.

The tamponade would be causing the intense discomfort Anna felt in her chest, and would have been the reason why she had felt such extreme anxiety. With every breath, the pressure in her chest would have worsened until she felt she could no longer catch her breath at all. She might have felt palpitations, her heart beating faster and in an irregular pattern, desperately trying to stop itself from drowning in the fluid-filled sac encasing it.

The external pacing box no longer worked, the silver needles inside her heart all but drowned in the bloody flood in her chest. Her heart rate careered away like wild horses spooked by the light of the moon.

The blood pressure monitor alarmed; finally it had recorded Anna's pressure. It read 50/30 mmHg. Anna was barely there. Classification of low blood pressure starts with a top-number reading of approximately 90 mmHg. Anna's was significantly below this. She now lay there not moving, her eyes rolled to the back of her head. She had stopped kicking and clutching at her chest. She almost looked as if she were sleeping.

The crash team arrived in less than five minutes. At that exact moment, Anna's heart rate plummeted on the screen. She was losing all cardiac output. There were long flat lines followed by a steep peak, a stomach-lurching drop, and then a mess of disorganized electrical activity. Her heart was generating electricity but no longer a pulse. It quivered inside its sac, blood-swamped, a gasping seabird stuck in an oily slick, the night never-ending, the sea black, the sky black, the blood darkening from lack of oxygen.

The rhythm Anna's heart had gone into was unshock-able. The crash team gathered around her. The source of the dangerous rhythm needed to be reversed, the blood drained from around her heart in order that it could contract again.

The cardiologist kept the ultrasound probe scanning her heart.

The crash team started CPR and secured an airway whilst the registrar and the SHO prepared to reopen Anna's chest. They needed to drain the blood and manually pump the heart from inside.

They were ready.

CPR was stopped.

The registrar used a scalpel, sliding the blade down the surgical incision they had made over a week ago. The SHO passed the registrar the wire cutters from the trolley, and he cut through the sternal wires holding Anna's chest together. The SHO suctioned the blood from around her heart so that they could see better. They pulled Anna's chest apart with clamps so that it would remain open and the registrar placed both his gloved hands deep inside, holding her heart between his palms and squeezing it to keep the blood circulating around her body.

He squeezed hard, his slippery hands pumping fast around the heart.

The crash team did a pulse check; there was still no pulse, and no blood pressure reading.

Somebody called out how long Anna had been without a pulse.

The registrar continued to squeeze her heart, trying to return her circulation and give her a pulse.

The time was eight minutes past midnight. Just eight minutes earlier, Anna had been on her hands and knees on the floor, but now everything had changed.

Her heart had stopped producing any electrical activity at all; it didn't spark and it didn't beat; it was totally empty of blood. Anna was dead.

24

Sometimes before somebody dies they get a sense it is going to happen. In nursing school we were taught about a symptom that often precedes a heart attack, a person experiencing a sense of impending doom. There is little known about this feeling, but it has been attributed to the pressure building up inside the chest from conditions such as Anna's cardiac tamponade. The feeling of low blood pressure could provide another explanation. Anna's blood pressure dropped rapidly, the blood barely running through the tributaries, and could have been the reason she knew before any of us that she was going to die.

The circulatory system consists of the heart, the blood and the blood vessels that branch out across the whole body. Circulation can be divided into two distinct net-works: the systemic circulation, which delivers oxygenated blood to organs and tissues and then travels back depleted to refuel and be sent out once more. And the pulmonary circulation, which carries dark blue blood to the lungs to be oxygenated and returns to the heart to start the cycle again.

The heart is protected by the thoracic cavity, the hard bones of the sternum and ribcage sheltering the soft pumping organ beneath. It has its own personal blood circulation, supplied by the coronary arteries that surround it. These vessels are renowned for becoming clogged with fatty deposits that can cause the vice-like grip of a heart attack.

Arching upwards from the left ventricle of the heart is the largest blood vessel we have: the aorta, a fat, flayed red-pepper vessel that pumps oxygen-rich blood away from the heart to organs and tissues around the rest of the body. It is in the wall of this vessel that a dangerous bulge, known as an aneurysm, can occur; if left untreated, it can swell to such a size that it ruptures, causing catastrophic bleeding beneath the surface and leading to almost instantaneous death.

Bleeding on the HDU is nearly always concealed like Anna's was, most often happening beneath the surface. We wait and watch for signs of it – a rise in venous pressure, a racing heart rate, quickened breath – but mostly are unable to see the blood as it pools in the hidden depths of the thoracic cavity, and have to rely on outward indications to detect the coming storm.

After shifts as a student nurse in the hospital on the hill, I walked from the medical wards to the birthing centre where my sister worked. Here I heard the guttural grunts and screams of women pushing their babies out into the daylight, and would stop mid corridor, startled by the sounds. I imagined the red splatter as the baby arrived, the warm puddle of blood beneath it, the umbilical cord still throbbing with life, the placenta delivered onto white hospital linen, a crimson eye staring up at the outside world it now belonged to. This blood affirmed life. It was on the hands of the midwives, streaked red on the legs of the mother, gathered in bright globs on the baby's fontanelle like sunspots.

Daisy had always wanted to be a midwife. At the hospital where she was training, she found the midwives were everything she had hoped they would be. They were kind, mysterious, full of knowledge, some of which had been learnt through years of experience, but some that was old and already known, like a glistening lode that ran right through them.

Daisy rang me after her first shift on the birth centre. She had seen her very first birth as a student midwife. I imagined her there, white lapels buttoned down and creases ironed into her sleeves just as Dad had taught us from his time spent ironing his uniform in the RAF.

The pregnant woman she was helping to look after was young and red-haired, and arrived on the birth centre out of breath and already in labour, being held up by her partner. Daisy's mentor, Karen, helped the woman into a room. As Daisy followed them in, another midwife whispered to them, 'Red for danger.' Karen waved her hand at her; Daisy didn't ask what she had meant.

They helped the woman onto a bed, where she clenched and unclenched her fists when the contractions came. As labour progressed, she started to writhe in pain, pulling at the edges of her nightie and roaring. Daisy described it as coming from deep within her. It was not distress, she explained, it was power.

My sister sat at the side of the room; she had been instructed to watch everything as it happened.

The woman's partner tried to tie her red hair back to keep it out of her face, but her head tossed from side to side. She held on to the metal headboard, her legs apart, her mouth a black 'O' pulling in air.

Karen saw the hair on the top of the baby's head. It was coming. She called in another midwife for the birth.

I could tell Daisy was smiling down the phone as she described the moment the baby was born, rushing out onto hospital linen on a wave of fluid. The air grew hot, and Daisy laughed as she went on to tell me how strange it was that there was now another person in the room.

The baby cried immediately. They kept the cord attached and passed her to the new mother, both of them pink and tear-streaked, relieved.

Karen, however, remained between the woman's legs, despite the baby being born. From her position behind her, Daisy could see that the midwife was totally still, as if feeling the direction of the breeze. Then she placed her arms either side of the bed and peered closely into the woman, her own body straight and tense, almost reverberating, as if sensing thunder yet to come.

In that exact moment, the woman began to bleed, fresh red blood gushing forth onto the bed. The second midwife pulled the emergency buzzer. Daisy said it was incredible how Karen had known what was normal and then, all of a sudden, what was not.

The woman continued to bleed. Daisy said it looked as

if she was losing pints of blood every minute, and she was in and out of consciousness.

The emergency team were on their way to the birth centre.

The woman was cannulated with wide-bore needles, intravenous fluids were run quickly through and blood was ordered from the blood bank: Code Red for haemorrhage. The blood was hot and red and still coming. Daisy could see it starting to clot on the sheets as it lay open to the air.

Karen remained between the woman's legs. Her latex gloves were now entirely red, her wrists and her arms red.

The woman had her eyes shut; her head lolled to one side. Her partner was helped out of the room by a support worker. He was covering his eyes with his hands.

The porter was running in with blood bags to transfuse.

The woman's new baby was safely resting on the Resuscitaire.

Karen said something to the other midwife, who nodded to her. Daisy watched in shock as she then pushed one hand into the woman's vagina, up as far as her wrist, placing the other on the woman's stomach to squeeze the uterus closed from the outside. Daisy later learnt this was called bi-manual compression: Karen was placing pressure on the vessels in the uterus to try and stop the bleeding herself.

It was agony for the woman. Her eyes opened immediately and she screamed in pain. She was too weak to move away, but she cried out and Daisy could barely watch.

There was blood everywhere. One of the midwives cradled the woman's head and whispered in her ear.

The emergency team arrived.

Drugs to get the uterus to contract and to slow the bleeding were given and more transfusions and fluids run through the cannulas in the woman's arm. There were people everywhere, drawing up drugs, hanging fluid bags, preparing to insert a urinary catheter; somebody else was writing the exact timings of observations and drugs being administered.

Slowly the woman's observations began normalizing. The oxygen mask misted as she took deep breaths and exhaled. Everything slowed down as the bleed came under control. The midwives and doctors in the room looked at the woman, their bloody gloved hands held up against their chests, watching as her circulation returned.

Afterwards, the midwives debriefed with a cup of tea in the staff room. It was here that Daisy met the midwife who had whispered to them as they'd entered the room before the birth. Her name was Mandy, and Daisy asked her what she had meant when she had said, 'Red for danger.'

Karen waved her hand again and told Daisy that she shouldn't take it too seriously, but there was a belief that women with red hair had a higher incidence of bleeding after giving birth.

Mandy said, 'I don't need it proved in any journal, Karen. We've seen it.'

Daisy listened to Karen and Mandy discuss the topic, two midwives who had both practised for nearly thirty years. Karen had raised her hands. 'Mandy, we want to teach our students best practice, up-to-date, evidence-based practice! Not full moons and red-haired women!'

No more was said on the subject as they finished their tea and Daisy and Karen went to write up their notes on the new mother, who now lay sleeping in clean sheets with her baby wrapped up beside her.

25

When I started working on the cardiothoracic HDU, I soon realized that not all our patients required open-heart surgery. Some patients arrived under the care of the cardiologists rather than the surgeons and were given medication or underwent tests and procedures to investigate and heal their hearts.

Mary was seventy-four years old and originally from Newcastle. She was transferred to our unit with all the symptoms of a heart attack: shortness of breath, chest pain, a rise in a particular cardiac enzyme, and changes on the electrocardiogram test we conducted. It revealed high rounded arches like tombstones on the ECG paper, suggesting that her heart muscle had not been receiving oxygen and had suffered an injury as a result. This injury was confirmed in her blood test, and Mary was hooked up to our monitors and treated on the heart attack protocol, given blood thinners, painkillers and medication to relax the walls of her vessels to allow the blood to pass more easily.

She had come in to A&E after experiencing a crushing heaviness on her chest in the early hours of the morning. She had called out for her husband and assumed he was using the toilet, but once she had broken through her sleep-headed twilight, she remembered that he had passed away only three weeks before.

She called an ambulance, wrapped a dressing gown around her and waited at the bottom of the stairs to be taken to hospital. She believed she was having a heart attack and turned off as many plug sockets as she could manage, then took her will from the drawer and placed it on the side table, just in case she wasn't going to return home.

By the time she came to us on the HDU, her chest pain was resolving but she was tired and her heart still flapped rapidly, a flock of birds disturbed by a thrown stone. She was looked after by the cardiologists and we kept her nil by mouth so that she could have an emergency angiogram to inspect the inside of her arteries for blockages.

This procedure involves the patient lying flat on a table surrounded by mobile X-ray screens. Local anaesthetic is applied to the skin around the wrist so that the doctor can insert a long, thin catheter tube up through the artery and guide it towards the heart. Patients are awake throughout this procedure, and whilst they don't describe it as painful, they say it feels as if there is a pushing beneath the surface of their skin.

Next, a contrast dye made from iodine is injected into the artery, making it possible for the X-ray scanner to see what is happening inside the vessels. On the screen, the hollows are illuminated and the branching arteries swirl with black, an ink stain spreading out across a white canvas.

Before the procedure, I checked on Mary regularly and recorded her observations on the chart. If her vessels proved particularly badly blocked, she might be listed for cardiothoracic bypass surgery. If they were fixable, the cardiology doctor might simply insert a stent to keep them open and keep the blood flowing through. If there was no blockage at all, it might just be that Mary needed to go home with new medication.

Home, as I found out, was in south London. She and her husband John had moved to the city twenty years ago to be closer to their children. Both she and John had grown up on the banks of the River Tyne, and left for the south on the day the Angel of the North statue was completed. John told his grandchildren that the statue had been erected in celebration of Mary, *his* angel of the north, since she had lived there all her life and the locals were sad to see her leave.

Mary told me they had been married for nearly sixty years and barely spent a day apart. When John was in the merchant navy, she went with him. At first the other sailors played tricks on him, mocking him for bringing his wife to sea, but after a week of high winds, Mary was seen at the bow of the ship putting the jackstaff back together whilst the sailors vomited over the side. From that day, the practical jokes stopped.

She had only been in hospital once before, when she broke her wrist a few years ago. It was the first time I heard her laugh all morning; it sounded like rainwater on tin, cold north-east rain trickling and tinkling down the copper wings of the angel.

She told me that one afternoon, she was tending to her roses in the garden. It was one of those clear blue summer days; the roses seemed to smell sweeter and the sheets on the line were dry within the hour. John was inside washing up whilst listening to the radio, the sounds drifting out down the garden path. She told me he always had it turned up extra loud because he was deaf as a doorpost and most of the time watched the way people's lips formed around words to help him hear.

Mary got up but lost her balance, her ankle rolling inwards and causing her to trip and fall. She landed badly on her wrist and took it in her other hand to see if it was broken. It certainly looked like it was: the bone stuck out awkwardly beneath the skin. Her head was spinning; she didn't think she could stand up. She shifted herself over away from the hard path and lay in the warm soil, staring up at her rose petals, pink and yellow scrims that let the sunshine through.

She called out for John. She called for him five or six times; craned her neck to see if he was coming. The radio still played, and occasionally she heard the clink of the dishes put out to dry on the draining board. John always took a long time to do the washing-up. It wasn't that there was a lot to do, but rather he liked to scrub them in hot water, let them dry a little and rinse off the remaining soap with fresh cold water before drying them by hand. Mary never understood why he did it that way; it was something that annoyed her and made her love him more. She thought of his soapy pink hands half submerged in the sink whilst she lay there.

She called again.

Nothing.

I listened to Mary, shocked that she had stayed outside in the garden so long with a broken wrist.

'I did,' she said. 'Early evening came and a few clouds passed above my head.' She laughed. 'The moon came out! But that bloody John didn't! He left me out there until it got cold, me and my poor broken wrist.'

'What happened?' I said.

'Well, I had a lot of time to think, as you can imagine. So I just lay back and thought of *us*, sixty years of us! How much time had passed. And do you know what? I laughed. Everything was funny when John was there.'

She sighed. 'He came out in the end. The poor thing looked sick with worry. He scooped me up – I was surprised at how strong he still was – and took me to A&E to get it X-rayed. It was broken after all.'

She looked down at her hands as they were now, at the cannula embedded beneath the skin, the starched bed linen stretched out across her legs.

'Gosh,' she said, and shook her head. 'What on earth am I going to do without him?'

I didn't say anything. I knew she was going to say more.

'Sixty years of us. And then that person is simply gone . . .'

'I'm so sorry,' I said. 'I can't even begin to imagine.'

'You know, when I woke up and John wasn't beside me, I spent the best part of an hour looking around the house for him: the toilet, the study, the living room. I even went out to the garden to see if he had wandered there. With the cancer being all over, I was always worried one day it would affect his brain.'

I nodded.

She shook her head. 'But he wasn't there. And then,

standing in the middle of the kitchen, I suddenly remembered he was dead. And that gave me such a fright. I'm not sure if it was because I had forgotten, or because he was gone, but I was terrified, about all of it.'

I held Mary's hand. We stayed like that for a while, and then the porter was standing in the doorway, smiling and making jokes about his cath-lab chariot, which he'd draped in a bed sheet, ready to take Mary for her procedure.

26

Downstairs in the cath lab, Mary had her surgical checklist reviewed and confirmed and a nurse took her observations. The lab was cool, everything silver and made from cold metal; it was how she might have imagined the foundations of the Angel to be: icy concrete interred metres beneath the ground in the rock below.

On the table, she was connected to an ECG machine and had her blood pressure and oxygen saturations set to record every fifteen minutes. A nurse reassured her that all the noise was just the lab team arranging the sterile equipment needed for the procedure. The nurse told Mary she would be with her at all times.

Mary's wrist was cleaned with a sterile scrub and then anaesthetized by the doctor, using a numbing medication delivered via a needle. He and the nurse guided a hollow tube through the skin and into the artery. Once it was in place, they removed the sharp from its innard so that they were left with a hollow straw-like instrument sitting inside the vessel. Now the cardiologist was passed the catheter that would travel to Mary's heart and began threading it through the artery.

Mary kept still on the table, her other hand gently drumming the hard surface beneath her in the tent-like quiet of the blue surgical blanket laid on top of her. Once the catheter was in place, the doctor told her that he would now be injecting the contrast dye into her vessels so that he could see them illuminated on the screen. If she liked, she could watch too. He turned a screen to face her.

The ink spread through her vessels, travelling down the sprawling branches, propelled by the soft pumping of her heart, contracting and expanding on the screen. The dye illuminated all her coronary arteries. There was no blockage, not a single one. The screen glowed in the dim light of the lab, a black ink stain frozen in time above the operating table. The doctor whispered something to the scrub nurse, who signalled for her colleague who was circulating the room to come and look.

A phone call was made.

A radiologist and another cardiac doctor arrived. They stared up at the screen, one narrowing his eyes, the other tilting his head to the side.

Mary had her own eyes closed, concentrating on her breathing whilst the team worked on her heart.

The radiologist pointed a long finger at the screen, tracing the shape he could see in the air before him like a child writing letters with a sparkler. The cardiologist took pictures of Mary's heart, the shape of it, the way it ballooned at the bottom, the left ventricle swollen and contracting feverishly to try and propel the blood around the bulge.

Back on the HDU with us, Mary lay against the pillows and rested her wrist on her lap. It had a compression band around it, inflated with air to stem the blood whilst it recovered from the angiogram. The cardiologists arrived and conducted an echocardiogram at the bedside, the lights dimmed, the blind pulled and Mary's heart brought to life on the screen.

Afterwards, the lead consultant sat down on the footstool beside the bed.

'Let me tell you the good news,' he said.

Mary sat up to talk to him. She cradled her wrist in her other hand.

'You haven't had a heart attack.'

Her brow furrowed. 'How can that be?' she said, putting her good hand up to her chest as if remembering the pain she'd experienced in the early hours.

'I know,' he said. 'It probably seems very strange.'

'Is it something worse?' she asked.

'Not necessarily,' the doctor replied. 'It's something quite unusual. Something I have seen before, but only once in my career.'

Mary tugged on her lower lip with her front teeth.

'It's called takotsubo cardiomyopathy.'

'Wow!' she said. 'Quite a mouthful. Tako . . .'

The doctor nodded. 'Yes,' he said. 'And you're quite right. It mimics all the symptoms of a heart attack. You did the right thing in treating it as such.'

'But it's not a heart attack?'

'No, we didn't find any blockages in your blood vessels. But the shape your heart has taken on is dangerous, and we need to make sure it returns to normal.'

'The shape?'

'Yes.' The doctor pulled a pen from his top pocket and a slip of paper from his trousers. 'Look, let me show you.' He nudged himself forward on the stool and began to draw.

Mary stared down at the paper.

'It looks like a vase? My heart looks like a vase?'

'Almost,' he said. 'Actually, takotsubo is the Japanese word for an octopus pot. Japanese fishermen would lay the heavy earthenware pot on the seabed and wait for an octopus to slide inside. When they pulled it up by its ropes, the octopus would be trapped inside the bulbous base, the neck too narrow for it to climb out and escape.'

'Gosh,' Mary said, momentarily distracted from news of her heart by the workings of the octopus trap.

The doctor continued. 'The shape of the pot is much like the shape your heart has taken on. Round at the base and skinny at the top, no good for a pump.'

'Why did this happen?' Mary said. 'Why did my heart change shape?'

'Well, Mary. That's something I was going to ask you. Has anything happened recently, a change in your home life, a stressor, a bereavement?'

Mary answered quickly. 'My husband has just died. Three weeks ago.'

The doctor didn't look away.

'I am so sorry,' he said.

'Thank you,' Mary replied. 'Why does it matter, for my heart?'

'Well, this condition is colloquially known as broken-heart syndrome.'

Mary's mouth hung open a little. 'Is that a joke?'

The doctor shook his head. 'It's not, I'm afraid. We have found that people who have suffered a trauma or a loss can exhibit all the signs of a heart attack, and yet when we look

162

inside, there are no indications of a heart attack having taken place. The organ has, however, changed shape, and this needs to be monitored as it impairs the pumping action and the flow of blood around your body.'

Mary nodded and sat back against the pillows, taking it all in.

'Broken-heart syndrome,' she sighed.

'I'm sorry,' the doctor said. 'You must have loved him very much.'

Mary smiled a little. She breathed out deeply.

'Yes,' she said. 'Sixty years of us.'

Before takotsubo cardiomyopathy was categorized in Japan in 1991, American scientists produced a study that explored the relationship between stress and damaged heart muscle.

In the lacustrine lowlands of Ohio, between peaceful glacial deposits and the lush Appalachian plateaus, two scientists spent time in the 1980s investigating nearly five hundred homicides that had taken place over the past thirty years in the area.

The victims they selected had all died from homicidal assault, but they focused in particular on fifteen victims who had not suffered internal injuries. Out of these fifteen, eleven were noted to have cardiac dysfunction evident in the muscle of the heart. This was despite having no internal bleeding or injury from the assault.

Furthermore, ten out of these fifteen victims had experienced some sort of confrontation or argument leading up to the physical assault. This drove the scientists to believe that stress hormones, such as adrenaline, had had a toxic effect on the heart cells.

Their theory was tested against a control. Fifteen fatalities from road traffic accidents were examined, but there was no trace of cardiac dysfunction in their hearts, as if the impact had rendered them dead instantaneously, with no opportunity for the body to become stressed or frightened and thus release adrenaline into the bloodstream.

The Mayans believed a soul could be displaced, wounded or even snatched from a living being, triggered by trauma or fright. They talked of winds stirring within a person, bones changing, blood speaking and jumping within the body when someone had experienced extreme fright.

Mary talked much about being frightened the night of the chest pain, frightened that she had forgotten John was dead, and terrified to be without him in the lonely house, short of breath as if something had been snatched from within her.

The Mayans believed the loss of a soul was dangerous, the various classes of soul viewed as the very essence of a person: their heart, their memory, their feelings instilled within them by ancient deities. The heart would often be plucked from the chest during sacrifice to appease supernatural beings that might covet the precious beating core. The Tzeltal Mayans from the highlands of south Mexico believed that the *ch'ulel*, the breath soul, resided in the blood and heart of a person, and that both the heart and the soul could be checked at the pulse.

*

For thousands of years, the heart has been a symbol of love and affection. Known as the centre of emotion by the ancient Egyptians and the Greeks, who similarly decided that the organ's central position in the body dictated its status, it was thought to be capable of harnessing great power.

It wasn't until the Roman Empire, however, that it became synonymous with feelings of love. The Romans, advised by Hippocrates, used the silphium plant to soothe their aches and pains. Its properties were used in cooking, and perfume was made from its blossom. They later discovered its role as a contraceptive. Thus the highly valued plant, with its heart-shaped seed pods, was stamped across Roman coins.

The image of a heart cleaved into two halves has long been recognized as a symbol of heartbreak, a lost love that has rendered the bearer lovesick, heavy-hearted and heartsore. I realized when I met Mary that this representation is not accurate at all; that the octopus-pot organ beating with three inky hearts nestled inside is a more truthful image.

The next weekend, Mary's heart was re-scanned by the cardiologists and was found to have almost completely returned to its normal shape.

'The octopus has gone?' she laughed as the cardiologist wiped the jelly from her chest.

'Almost,' he smiled. 'Are you feeling well in yourself?'

'Much better,' she said.

'Then I think we'll send you home. You're going to

have to take some medication with you, and we'd like to see you again in clinic in six weeks' time. Any more symptoms, come straight back to us.'

'I will, Doctor,' Mary said.

'Who will be at home with you?' the doctor asked.

At this, Mary smiled. 'My children are coming to collect me,' she said. 'We're going to go back home, up north for a couple of weeks. We're going to show the grandchildren John's angel on the top of the hill.'

The doctor nodded and took Mary's hand in his own. Her pulse was powerful beneath the skin.

27

To examine the way blood flows through the body, the nurse must complete an assessment of circulation, using the technique of 'look, listen and feel'. It is important to recognize how well filled up with blood a patient is in order to understand how well perfused their organs and tissues are.

During assessment of circulation it is fundamental that all elements of the examination are completed, including measuring blood pressure, heart rate, capillary refill, limb temperature and sometimes urinary output. Looking at a person's colour can give a quick indication that blood volume has been lost, or that haemoglobin, the oxygen-carrying component of red blood cells, is running low.

The human body has an overall circulating blood volume of four to five litres, equivalent to almost ten pints. When blood is lost, a person may rapidly descend into shock, their body desperately compensating to try and function despite losing volume.

A person can lose 20 per cent of their whole-blood volume before starting to become symptomatic, by which point the deterioration into hypovolaemic shock may be rapid and irreversible. Hypovolaemic shock is classified as a depletion in volume so that circulation can no longer be supplied to the rest of the body and its tissues. This kind of loss can be caused by vomiting or diarrhoea, obvious injury or wounds. The bleeding can, however, be less obvious, concealed in abdominal or thoracic cavities, in a tear of the aorta or from fractured bones deep below muscle and fat. Fracture of the femur can cause over a litre and a half of hidden blood loss. This quantity will soon manifest symptoms: a significant drop in blood pressure, a heart rate climbing high above the blood pressure, marked on the chart like a full moon rising, forecasting a turbulent night ahead.

This increase in heart rate is caused by the heart desperately trying to fight back against the low circulating volume with a more vigorous pumping mechanism, attempting to drive round what little blood is left in the body. At first the pulse may be described as 'full' or 'bounding', a new pup let off the lead, leaping forth across the riverbank to get to the other side. But soon, as the body continues to lose volume, the pulse tires and becomes weak or thready, and eventually hard to feel at all beneath the fingertips. A pulse is generated by the stretchy arterial walls throbbing as the heart contracts, causing a pressure wave that can be felt at various pulse points through the body: the wrist, the neck, the groin. Analysing a pulse – from the Latin *pulsus*, 'to beat' – proves a useful indication of how much blood is being pumped from the heart and driven around the body, and at what strength. The pulse can be counted, telling us how fast or slow the heart is beating and whether that heartbeat is irregular.

Whilst nurses often use their fingers to feel for a pulse, electronic cardiac monitors are able to detect pulse using the pulse oximeter attachment. This is a small finger-worn device that uses red infrared light absorption to calculate how much oxygen is in the blood, and in addition measures the pulsing arterial blood to determine a beat. There are, however, limitations to the device, especially during the stages of hypovolaemic shock. If the person has lost a significant amount of fluid, their fingers may have grown cold, peripherally shut down with all the blood vessels constricted in order to conserve what is left. They might be lying in their hospital bed shivering, warm blood no longer surging within them. With shivering, the infrared light is unable to take a clear reading of either oxygen level or pulse, and more invasive techniques will need to be used.

The nurse must also assess blood pressure, using either a blood pressure cuff or invasively using an arterial line inserted by a doctor: a long, thin plastic tube sitting inside an artery that provides a waveform deciphered on the screen alongside a numerical blood pressure reading. Neither blood pressure nor heart rate readings are good early indicators of shock, since the body uses its natural defence mechanisms to adapt, thus exhibiting barely any change in cardiovascular state.

Dad's aortic valve was severely narrowed, preventing blood from flowing through his body. Whilst it was one of the most common valve diseases, it was also the most serious. Survival rates without treatment for severe symptomatic aortic stenosis are low: 50 per cent of people will be alive within two years and only 20 per cent survive at five years without an aortic valve replacement.

We didn't know how long Dad's valve had been diseased, but the symptoms he was having – shortness of breath and fainting at the table – indicated that it had progressed to an advanced stage and needed surgery urgently.

Like Mary, he underwent a coronary angiogram at the hospital I worked in to see whether the vessels supplying his heart would also need fixing. The test revealed that three of the main arteries supplying the heart with blood were 70 per cent blocked. He would need an aortic valve replacement and a triple bypass under the cardiothoracic team.

On the ward, Mum unpacked Dad's belongings, placing them neatly in the bedside drawers, and we all kissed him goodnight. We would see him the next morning; he was first on the list for his open-heart operation.

Disability

Don't shoot for the stars, we already know what's
there. Shoot for the space in between because
that's where the real mystery lies.

Vera Rubin, astronomer

28

During Dad's admission for cardiac surgery, he spent time on the heart-lung machine, his blood taken from the right side of his heart and pumped extracorporeally through plastic tubing, where it curved round spinning rollers and whisked through lung-like filters until it returned to him, oxygenated, bright red and changed.

Once he was wheeled into theatre, we went home and waited for the surgery to finish. I imagined Dad laid out on the operating theatre table. He'd had an arterial line and central venous catheter inserted into his wrist and neck, and had been put to sleep, a long breathing tube slithered down his throat whilst somebody taped his eyes shut.

I knew the surgeon who would be leading Dad's bypass and valve operation; he had conducted one of the first cardiothoracic operations I had ever watched, before I started on the HDU. At that time I had never seen his full face; it was hidden beneath a surgical mask and I could see only his eyes, scanning the open chest beneath him, the gold initials on the arms of his glasses catching the light. That morning I stood on a footstool, leaning above the patient with just the surgical blue drape, a sterile barrier between patient and surgeon, separating us. There was nothing to hold on to for balance, and standing for five hours on a small stool, rocking back and forth to take the weight off my feet, I had to make sure I didn't grab at something nearby that would bring the operation clattering to a standstill.

Back at home, we waited for news. I imagined the surgeon as he made a long, clean incision down Dad's chest; it was the same chest that rose above the water beneath a summertime sun, soaring, arms arced over his shoulders before crashing through the surface, lake water curling at the edges. I closed my eyes and thought of him, all white splash and breath, there one minute, gone the next.

I imagined somebody adjusting the light above the surgeons, the handle covered with a sterile cover. Dad's sternum would then be laid bare, flayed, a flat limestone ridge that jutted out from his thoracic cavity. The surgeon would be able to cut through it easily with a serrated saw, his registrar helping to prise Dad's chest open with stainless-steel retractors that he held in place, his forearm quivering with the task.

Dad's heart would still be beating, his lungs still puffed up, full of air, ready to breathe, ready to tell us a joke.

The surgeons would then start to remove the vessels they needed for bypass.

The anaesthetist would administer a blood-thinning medication and wait until the clotting time was correct before connecting Dad to the heart-lung machine.

The clock on the wall would not make a sound.

In the corner of the room, the perfusionist might check her machine again. The tubing would be filled with over two litres of electrolyte solution in readiness for Dad's blood, which would soon come and mix with her own cool, sterile liquid.

Only her roller pump would disturb the quiet.

The consultant would plumb wide tubing into Dad's heart and place a clamp across his aorta to stop the blood flowing into the chambers. Cold potassium would be injected to stop it beating. His heart would then be empty.

The surgeons would start the grafts first, taking time to stitch the new vessels to the coronary arteries to avoid the blockages. They would work quickly. Dad's heart would be completely still in his chest.

When the bypass was complete, they would replace his heart valve, removing the diseased valve and the brittle calcium deposits surrounding it, which were at risk of travelling in his bloodstream to his brain.

I imagined the scrub nurse holding her sterile-gloved hands interlaced and close to her chest as if in prayer, waiting to pass the next piece of equipment.

When the new valve was in place, they would release the clamp across Dad's aorta. Within seconds his heart would begin to beat, squirming until it remembered how to contract. The surgeons would check that everybody was happy with Dad's observations, that his heart rate, rhythm and blood pressures could manage without the machine. The bypass machine would be weaned from his body, the pipes taken out, chest drains and pacing wires inserted and stainless-steel wires used to close his breastbone. He would then be stitched back together, the skin closed over the new heart valve and pumping vessels. I had heard patients back on the ward refer to themselves as part of the Zipper Club, the long white scar down their chests forever reminding them that they had once been unzipped and then put back together again after receiving open-heart surgery.

Afterwards Dad would be taken to Cardiac Recovery, where he would remain intubated for the night, a tube down his throat breathing for him. The consultant would check on him. The anaesthetist would fiddle with the dials on the ventilator, making sure he was getting enough oxygen. I knew the nurses would be titrating the doses of his infusions, ensuring that his heart was pumping force-fully, that he had enough volume inside his body to maintain good blood pressures, keeping all his organs nicely filled up and working, and that he was comfortably sedated, unaware of what was going on around him.

We all decided we didn't want to see him whilst he was still sedated, and spent a sleepless night at home thinking of him lying in the cold, low-ceilinged hum of Cardiac Recovery, his blue eyes taped closed, his mind temporarily unmoored from its stem whilst it drifted away in anaesthe-tized dreams, somewhere far away that we couldn't reach.

We visited him the following afternoon. He was sitting up in his chair, breathing for himself, attached to the car-diac monitor with ECG electrodes. He had a red arterial cannula in his wrist, providing a constant measurement of his blood pressure, and a long central cannula in his neck that measured his venous pressure and drip-fed him fluids and medication to keep his heart pumping well. A long white strip of plaster down his chest covered the closed surgical wound and the bruised skin beneath. In his side he had three chest drains stitched in place. I fol-lowed the garden-hose tubing looping out from beneath his gown and down into plastic bottles collecting his blood. The nurses had attached the bottles to the suction unit on the wall to assist drainage of the fluid gathered around his operation site.

Mum sat with Dad, holding his hand. He kept falling asleep, his head resting against the hard-backed chair. He was still on a morphine drip. When he woke and looked around the room, his eyes were pale like moonstones; you could barely see the pupils, and he gazed at his surroundings as if he had no memory of being brought here at all.

Mum had found a Harris Tweed hat in the woods near the house where Dad used to walk me to school. Harris Tweed was Dad's favourite type of tweed, a hand-woven herringbone pattern dyed and spun in the remote Outer Hebrides of Scotland. He collected tweed jackets and trawled charity shops for interesting designs and colours. I had brought the hat into Cardiac Recovery and now pulled it down neatly on Dad's head. It smelt of rain and wet ferns. He looked more like himself, setting off to walk the dog in the woods on a damp Monday morning. He didn't notice I'd put the hat on him.

In Cardiac Recovery, patients can range from being completely sedated using medication to awake and aware of their surroundings. Dad was somewhere in between. He had recently been woken up and had the tube removed from his throat, but the remnants of the medication were still in his bloodstream. The unit had ten beds and looked after any patients who had undergone cardiac surgery, both elective and emergency. Whilst one patient might have had a valve and vessels replaced, like Dad, another might have had a tear in one of their major arteries sewn back together, or been stabbed late one evening and needed a chest drain inserted.

There are many causes of delirium in the post-operative cardiac patient. These can include medication sensitivities, dehydration, lack of sleep, electrolyte disturbances, infection and low oxygen levels in the blood. Dad's electrolytes needed topping up frequently, pocket-sized packets of potassium hooked up to the drip in his neck. He didn't sleep: the nurses tried to persuade him to wear the tight oxygen mask overnight to keep his lungs open, as the oxygen in his blood was dangerously low. To help with his delirium, we were told to bring in items that would remind him of home: photos or letters, a clock or calendar to reorientate him. He had a watch with a threadbare leather strap. Mum brought it in and attached it to his wrist. Immediately he slid the strap around so that the gold face sat upwards on the inside of his wrist, as he did at home. He glanced down to look at it. He remembered that part of himself at least.

Dad wouldn't remember any of his time spent in Cardiac Recovery. He was sleepy and disorientated, but his heart was pumping well. After one night, he was moved upstairs to the HDU where I worked. I had taken a week off; I didn't want to try to look after other people whilst he was recovering.

I stared at the big paper chart marking his progress that was clipped beside his bed. The nurses were monitoring his level of consciousness after the operation since he was still sleepy and disorientated. They had turned off his morphine drip despite still having the discomfort of the drains in his chest, because they had noted that his pupils were too small and he wasn't able to tell them where he was, even with prompting.

They had scored him using the Glasgow Coma Scale, a tool devised in the 1970s to provide a practical way of assessing impaired consciousness in a person. It is one of many tools used to assess consciousness and is divided into three sections, allowing the nurse to examine what kind of stimulation the patient requires in order to elicit a response from them. The three sections are related to eye-opening, speech and movement. The highest a person can score is fifteen, indicating that they are able to open their eyes spontaneously, are orientated to time, place and person, and can obey commands such as lifting an arm or a leg when asked to do so.

Dad was scoring fourteen out of fifteen. He wasn't able to remember which hospital he was in, but he could remember that he had had a heart operation. He kept asking whether the doctors had put his heart back once they had finished. The nurses assured him that they had, and that they could see it beating on the screen. They pointed upward and Dad followed their fingers with his eyes as if looking at the night sky, watching the rhythm of his heartbeat unfurl like a meteor trail across the black screen. They told him that he was doing well; to keep drinking, to keep deep-breathing. They told him to hold himself firmly around the chest when he coughed, like a tight hug; to imagine he was holding Mum and never wanting to let her go.

29

In the disability section of the ABCDE examination, the nurse begins a neurological assessment of the patient. This consists of investigating the degree of brain dysfunction impacting upon a person's state of consciousness, looking for the source and how to rectify the problem. A person exhibiting an altered state of consciousness might have a head injury or severely low blood sugar; they might have undergone surgery or have such pain that they are unable to function as before. Their disability could present as pupils reacting sluggishly to light, a slurred voice or rigid, stiffened limbs stretched out and clenched against the bed sheets as a result of a seizure.

Before assessing a person's consciousness, the nurse must ensure that all preceding parts of the ABCDE examination are stable. They must check that the airway is safe and that all reversible causes that could have decreased the person's cognition are excluded. For instance, if the person's breathing has been deemed abnormal in the breathing part of the examination, it may be that their level of consciousness has deteriorated due to not enough oxygen travelling to their brain. The nurse needs to concentrate on the breathing section to fix the problem, applying oxygen, taking arterial blood, ensuring a chest X-ray is ordered and making sure the medical team are aware of the worsening condition of the patient and will come and review them immediately.

Dad's blood gas was acidotic. He was storing too much carbon dioxide in his body since his lungs were not able to fully inflate. He needed to wear the breathing mask that would force air into his lungs, but because he was confused, he was uncompliant. The surgeons came to speak to him, but he didn't retain the information. The nurses sat with him and explained over and over again, their eyes momentarily drifting up to the monitor that showed his oxygen levels dipping dangerously low.

The ABCDE assessment can move fluidly through A–E as required, a pendulum rocking back and forth between physical examinations until the nurse feels each problem is stable and under control. It may be that by the time they are ready to reassess disability, the person's consciousness has improved as a result of treating a problem in a previous section. Then again, it might be that the problem is located in the brain and nervous system and therefore an assessment of disability should be fully explored.

The brain can be affected by numerous internal and external sources. Low oxygen levels, imbalanced electrolytes, tumours, swelling and bleeding can impact upon the way we think, speak, move and understand the world around us. Head trauma from falling objects, after-dark punches or road traffic accidents may render a person unconscious through severe injury to the brain, despite its hard skull casing.

Our brains are soft, made up of a wrinkled jelly-like mass of protein and fat and split into two halves, which can easily be deciphered on the black-and-white screen of a CT scan. The midline, often presented as a glowing white ghostly wisp down the centre of the brain, can shift abnormally to one side after severe injury. This clinical picture, known as a midline shift, carries an extremely poor prognosis for the patient, their very self displaced across a border and unable to go back.

Inside the brain there is a sprawling constellation of nerve cells, billions of electrical stalks that transmit information and messages through the nervous system, a grid-like circuit lit up by the sparking of ideas, thoughts and sensations, the glowing trails of feeling flashing and flitting through the body. Despite this spectacle of lights, the brain is shrouded in darkness. Scientists have studied it for thousands of years and are still not able to illuminate its capabilities fully. In particular, the question of how we perceive the world around us and transform our electrochemical signals into conscious experience is one yet to be answered.

The universe is similar to our brains. Space contains a strikingly comparable amount of galaxies as our brains do neurons. Grey matter in the brain has approximately six billion neurons within it; the cerebellum houses almost sixty-nine billion. Our observable universe consists of one hundred billion galaxies, made up of swirling dust and gas clouds, black holes, exploding stars and drifting dark matter that, much like the brain, we still struggle to fully understand. As a child, I was fascinated by outer space and stuck endless glow-in-the-dark stars across my bedroom ceiling. When I became a nurse, I realized that the brain was similarly mysterious and uncharted, and it was on the night shifts that we saw the depths of its impenetrable dark.

Astronomers and astrophysicists discuss the observable universe. That is to say, there are places beyond it that we cannot see, record or measure. Despite having access to billions of galaxies within our own glittering sphere, we are not yet able to gauge the depth of what exists beyond the edges of the observed. In the same way, while the brain has been dissected and lit up, scanned, stained and probed to find answers, still mystery pervades. There are parts of the brain, such as those that experience consciousness, that exist beyond our current knowledge, unexplored, unobserved matter drifting beyond our grasp.

As nurses, we can assess level of consciousness quickly using a tool well recognized in emergency and trauma settings. The AVPU scale provides an immediate gauge of a person's state of consciousness. AVPU stands for alert, voice, pain, unresponsive, and measures at what grade of stimulus the patient is responding: are they alert, or responding only to voice or pain, or are they entirely unresponsive, no longer aware of the universe around them.

A patient who is alert will likely be sitting up in bed and possibly able to talk back. This is not to say they are not unwell, nor that what they are saying can be comprehended, but for the moment their eyes are open and they are conscious, breathing and responding; they are able to keep their airway open by themselves.

A patient who only responds to voice may present as drowsy. They may be intoxicated, or curled up on their side from an overdose; they may not have enough oxygen circulating to their brain, or they may have received a trauma to the head that has impacted upon their ability to stay awake. At this point, they only rouse when their name is called; other than that, their eyes are closed and they appear to be sleeping.

A person who doesn't respond to voice might only be woken up when pressure or pain is applied to them. This usually takes the form of a trapezius pinch, firm pressure applied to the patient's shoulder in the form of a squeeze, to try and elicit a response. If a patient doesn't respond to the painful stimulus, they are deemed unresponsive; if they are unresponsive and not breathing, immediate cardiopulmonary resuscitation is commenced. Their heart might have stopped and it is now a life-threatening emergency, a crash call, hands on chest and defibrillator charged and ready to go.

If the patient who is unresponsive is still breathing for themselves, they are placed on their side in the recovery position and the team must work hard to investigate the reason why they are critically unwell. Blood will be drawn and brain scans ordered; a patient history needs to be obtained from friends or family to try and see if there were any preceding causes as to why this person now lies in a hospital bed unresponsive, unconscious and unaware of their surroundings, their consciousness entirely altered.

30

My first experience of looking after someone with an altered state of consciousness was as a student nurse five years earlier. I had seen on my placements what an important role the healthcare assistants played in the hospital, and decided to work a shift on the weekend in this role to get some extra income and to see whether the neurology wards would be an interesting place to work when I qualified.

The neuro wing was made of glass and steel. The ward was on the top floor. I travelled up in the windowless silver lift, staring at my own reflection, imagining the world outside. I was nervous: I had never been to this ward and hadn't worked with patients who had neurological conditions before. In my mind I rose up past the sycamore trees in the park with their translucent helicopter seeds pirouetting to the ground, up past the traffic rushing along the main road. I looked down on the baked yellow brick of the hospital entrance in the morning sun, the wrapped-up dressing-gowned patients pushing crystalline drips and smoking cigarettes outside the old wing.

The ward was one member of staff short, and so there were thirty-one patients and four nurses. There were only two members of support staff on duty that day: myself and another healthcare assistant.

I watched the day staff take notes in the empty boxes

on their handover sheets, using different-coloured pens or asterisks to remind themselves which patients were on antibiotics or specialist infusions; which were having procedures today and therefore had to be kept nil by mouth; which were end-of-life and needed to be made comfortable; and which were scoring highly on the warning charts, indicating that they would need more attention and possible escalation to a higher dependency.

I stared at the neurology abbreviations; they meant little to me. I had no time to ask anyone for clues, as the patients needed to be helped with their breakfasts.

The nurses started their medication rounds, filing out from the staff room to collect drug trolleys and computers. I watched them wheel the trolleys across the linoleum, their faces screen-lit, glasses hooked in their tunics, their minds full of invisible to-do lists. They gave out tablets to the people who were able to put out their hand and recite their name and date of birth so that the nurse could check she was giving the right tablets to the right person.

Next the nurse would go to the patients who needed their tablets administered via their feeding tubes. I was filling up a papier-mâché bowl of warm water, about to start a patient wash. The other healthcare assistant was in another bay with the curtains drawn, helping somebody else.

The nurse put the brakes on the drug trolley and smiled at me as she crushed tablets in a little yellow pill pot, grinding the top and bottom together so that a tiny puff of white dust wisped away when she opened it.

'I won't be long,' she said. 'And once I'm done, I'll help you with Liam.'

I looked at the patient I was due to wash.

'I might be okay,' I said.

The nurse smiled again. She dropped the crushed tablets into sterile water, stirred, then drew up the cloudy mixture in a syringe to push into Liam's feeding tube.

'Morning, Liam,' she said. 'Just giving you your anti-seizure medication, some painkillers and an antibiotic. It's a delicious cocktail,' she added. 'Your favourite, actually, your mum said. A mojito. I haven't got one of those little cocktail umbrellas, though, unfortunately.'

She flushed the feeding tube with more sterile water, took off her gloves and apron, washed her hands and waved goodbye to us both, drawing the blue curtain around as she left.

'See ya in a bit!' I heard her call out as she moved into the next bay.

I was alone with Liam. I held the bowl of water in front of me, ready to place on the table. Liam's head had been resting to one side whilst the nurse administered his medication, softly placed against the pillow as if he was sleeping. She had been able to push the medication through his feeding tube without waking him.

He was awake now and turned to look at me, and it was then that I saw he was missing half of his head. I heard myself gasp. Liam didn't seem to notice my surprise; he looked around the room but his eyes didn't rest on anything in particular. He had deep brown eyes, almost black, as if the pupil and the iris were mixed from the same carob pigment, like staring into a black hole without stars.

'Morning, Liam,' I said quickly. 'My name's Molly, I'm going to help you with a wash this morning. Is that okay?'

He didn't speak. I couldn't be sure if he had heard me at all. He raised both arms and extended them away from his body. On his hands he wore white cotton boxing gloves strapped around his wrists with Velcro ties. They were safety mittens, used to stop him from pulling at his feeding tube, his intravenous cannula, his urinary catheter or anything else that he needed to keep him well in hospital. He banged the soft boxing glove against the side of his head that was still intact.

On the other side, where his skull was missing, his head was concave, a deep, smooth curve like a bowl. His scalp and hair had been stretched and stapled to cover the sunken hollow; he had thick dark hair like a shoe-shine brush, black eyebrows that joined in the middle, sitting above his black-hole eyes.

'Let's get you freshened up,' I said. 'We'll be quick, and then cover you back up, keep you nice and warm.'

Liam didn't look any older than me. He had neatly trimmed stubble on his chin and above his lip, but his cheeks were smooth. He must have had family, as in his locker was a shaver and aftershave, an expensive cologne and lip balms and moisturizers in a zipped bag.

I had a look through them. He had the same toiletry bag as my dad. I imagined Dad's one sitting beside the mirror in our family home, the same striped bag I had seen sitting there for years. I thought of the way our bathroom smelt after Dad had showered, entirely different from me or my sister or mum. The air was almost medicinal, antiseptic and mint. Dad's bathroom bag was packed with cheap disposable razors; we could never understand how he finished a shave unscathed. He had talcum powder that hung in the air after a shower like early-morning snowfall.

I squeezed some of Liam's shower gel into the bowl, wetted some hospital wipes and arranged a towel just below his neck.

'Here,' I said, placing the warm wipe against his cheek so as not to frighten him. I wasn't sure if he knew I was there.

Liam gazed at me, his eyes fixed on mine. I tried not to look at the dent in his head, the softness of his scalp stretched so taut it seemed to pulsate.

'Are you okay in there?' A voice from outside.

'We're okay,' I said, although I felt glad of the company.

'Need a hand?' It was the other healthcare assistant, who had come to find me.

'That might be good,' I said.

Liam thrashed his boxing glove mitts against the side of the bed.

'Okay, okay,' the healthcare assistant said, tying a gown around her waist. 'Hiya, Liam,' she said, and stroked the good side of his head. 'It's Sammy, the one that's always washing you in freezing tap water,' she laughed.

Liam looked at her, then rested his head back against the pillow. He appeared calmer now that she was here.

When we had finished helping Liam to wash, I asked Sammy what had happened to him, how he had lost one side of his head.

'Aren't you a nursing student?' she said, grinning at me.

I hadn't said I was, but I nodded anyway.

'Not done neuro before, have you?'

I shook my head.

'He's a craniectomy.' She tapped her own skull with her pen. 'The docs have removed a flap of bone in his skull to let it swell upwards instead of down. If it swells down, you're pretty much dead,' she said bluntly. 'Come with me . . .'

We left Liam and I followed her into the clinical room, where there was a laminated drawing of a brain and an upside-down skull on the wall.

'The docs tell me everything.' She smiled at me. 'See here?' She pointed at the bottom of the skull, where there was a dark hole for the spinal cord to pass through. 'Well, if they don't let the brain swell up and out, it might swell downwards and slurp out of the bottom of that hole like a Mr Whippy.'

I stared at her, then back at the black hole in the base of the skull.

'Removing that flap of skull saved Liam's life. He'll probably get better than how he is now, when the swelling goes down a bit, once they've removed all the blood clots around his brain . . .'

'He will?' I said.

She nodded. 'Probably. His mum wants to take him to a neuro rehab in Hertfordshire so that they can all be closer to home.'

'What happened to him?' I asked.

'Poor boy. I've got a son his age,' Sammy replied. 'Liam was a delivery driver. You remember the storm just a few months ago?'

'Yeah,' I said.

'Well, he got out of his van because his swipe card wasn't opening the parking barrier at the depot. It looked like the barrier had jammed in some way, but he managed to loosen it, tried his swipe card again and this time the pole went up. As he was turning to get back in the van, the wind – you know, it was like a hundred miles an hour – swung the pole so that it dropped smack-bang on the front part of his head.' She pointed at the top of her own forehead. 'I think that's why he can't speak at the moment; the front part of his brain was affected.'

I stared at the poster on the wall, the multicoloured lobes and the gaping skull.

'Come on then, let's get on with these washes. You do Bed Three and I'll meet you at Bed Six to help her together.'

'Okay,' I said and walked back into the bay. I couldn't believe it wasn't even nine o'clock yet, and I had another eleven hours to go. I went over to the sink to get another bowl of warm water. Liam was sitting upright, staring out of the window with his big black equine eyes. The morning sunlight fell on his face. I wondered if he could feel it.

31

Over the next few days, Dad was moved to the main ward. His confusion had improved, but something else had replaced the hallucinations.

He said that he no longer felt like himself, as if his body remained tethered to the bed by drains and tubes, cardiac leads and wires, whilst his mind, fuzzy at the edges, drifted to the other side of the room, where it sat and watched the workings of the day. He felt slow, disconnected, unable to align himself with the person he had been before his blood was drawn out towards a whirring centrifugal cylinder beneath the bright operating theatre lights, and forced back again in a different form.

It was almost as if he had undergone an out-of-body experience. This phenomenon is well documented but not yet completely understood.

Researchers have suggested that during bypass surgery, and time spent 'on the pump', fractals of fatty plaques, blood clots, bubbles and even minuscule shards of debris from the heart-lung machine itself can be released into the patient's bloodstream, altering the make-up of their circulation, damaging its integrity, looping back towards them with dangerous flotsam and jetsam in the river of their blood. Perhaps a plaque from an old pulmonary moraine carved off and travelled to Dad's brain, or a bubble popped on its way through his carotid arteries, damaging the flow of blood. However, similar changes have been noted in people suffering with cardiovascular disease who have not been operated on; perhaps the altered state of mind is a product of the condition, rather than the time spent on the pump.

Either way, Dad felt different.

One afternoon during visiting hours, I held his hand. He had had his chest drains taken out, the central line into his vena cava and arterial line removed and his wounds re-dressed. He had spent a long extra week in hospital trying to get his bladder to function normally, but was kept on the main ward, which meant he could walk around, no longer tied to the bed by monitoring leads.

He was recovering well, but spent a lot of time ordering his thoughts, watching the world pass by in the chink of corridor he could see through the open doorway. He said the whole hospital came to life in that bustling aperture, almost like a film set.

Junior doctors hurried past with stethoscopes draped round their necks like wilting blooms, blood gas syringes twizzled between their fingers, hoping the blood wouldn't clot before they reached the analyser. Nurses rattled by with clunking metal cupboards on wheels, drug trolleys, laptops, blood pressure machines, black leather soles leaving scuff marks on the floor. Porters whizzed past, speedy hospital gurneys with patients wired up from chest to wrist, portable monitors flashing red as they were taken through the HDU swing doors, where Dad had come from a week ago. He liked watching patients walk past – if they were slower than him – some carefully clutching groin drains, or catheter bags bulging with sunflower-yellow urine, or chest drains in their lantern-shaped bottles, sloshing with luminous serous fluid, held up as if searching for new land.

Much of his time was spent lying in bed waiting to go home. He was in a bay of two beds and had become friendly with a younger man who had had the same heart operation. This man had four daughters and was keen to get back to his job working on the London Underground. He said that since having the pipework of his veins and arteries re-routed, he would never be able to look at the tortuous coloured lines of the Tube map in the same way. He was soon discharged with no complications, and the paper curtain was now half drawn around an elderly Asian patient with lots of family visiting, bringing food in lunch boxes.

That afternoon with me, Dad cried when he talked about his mum. He had lain there in the quiet of the hospital at night, thinking of her, the memory so vivid he couldn't be sure she wasn't there, standing in the gloom of the doorway looking after him. Since the operation, his mind was showing him things in a whole new way.

'She always said that the friends she made at the hospital were unlike any friends she ever had again,' he said. 'The fun she had with her nurses on the night shift was something she yearned for when she no longer worked.' He wiped at his nose. 'It was a sacred time in some low-lit, whispered way . . . I think it was hard for her to describe; even harder to be without it.'

Dad said he had lain there and listened to the sounds of the nurses on the ward all night, young, straight out of nursing school, giggling together, whispering, their footsteps back and forth a comfort in the enveloping dark.

32

Dad's post-operative state was the result of a number of factors. He had spent a long time on the heart-lung machine, he had not received enough oxygen in the hours afterwards, he hadn't opened his bowels, he had a chest infection, he hadn't slept, and the electrolytes in his blood were out of balance.

It was as a student nurse on a placement with the London Ambulance Service that I first learnt about the effect chemical imbalances have on the brain.

We were called at nine thirty in the morning to our first job. It was a blue-skied spring day; a smudge of blackbirds flew across Waterloo Road heading towards the gardens by the Thames. Ryan, the paramedic, and I had our windows open and could smell hot pastry and meat fillings drifting out from the pasty counter in the station. Ryan stuck his head out and breathed in deeply, eyes closed.

I looked at him.

'I haven't had any breakfast,' he said, laughing at himself.

The radio bleeped. Ryan tuned in. A tinny voice from the emergency operating centre spoke to us:

'Thirty-year-old male at Brightside Brain Injury Unit, patient breathing but unresponsive.'

Ryan pressed '1' to say we were en route to attend.

Brightside Brain Injury Unit was five miles away, but with the blue lights on, we would be there in under ten minutes. Ryan belted himself in, reversed the truck, checked his mirrors and pulled out onto the busy Waterloo Road, switching the blue lights and sirens on. We were off.

People stared up at us as we weaved through the traffic. I tried to keep my eyes straight ahead. Ryan sang along to the radio as his eyes darted from rear-view to wing mirror. A couple saw us hurtling towards them and held each other back at a zebra crossing. A schoolchild holding her mother's hand let it go and plugged her ears with her fingers. Inside the truck, it wasn't so loud, though the gurney in the back shook in its brackets, and some electrodes from the ECG machine dangled from the shelf, moving back and forth in sync like river reeds swaying beneath the water.

'Been here before?' Ryan looked over at me.

'Never.' I shook my head. 'I've not had any neuro placements yet.'

'We get called out here a bit. They have great carers but only a few trained nurses on the floor, and if somebody gets sick, there's only so much they can do at the unit before having to call us in. They know the residents really well, so that's always helpful when taking a history from them.' He looked at the radio. 'To be honest, I'm surprised we didn't get more information from the EOC. Maybe it's a new resident that they don't know so much about.'

Ryan went on to explain that the unit was a residential home looking after people who had experienced a brain injury or who had a neurological condition and required support with their everyday needs. It could look after twenty-five residents at one time and also offered rehabilitation in order to help get people back home.

As we neared the unit, a few white puffs of cloud hung loosely in the sky as if gathered to see what was going on. We parked in the ambulance spot and picked up the gear. It was heavy on my shoulder.

Inside, a woman at the desk signalled us upstairs and then swivelled her chair back to the computer screen and her cup of tea.

Four care workers wearing purple tabards were waiting for us, looking nervous. One of them was crouched beside a man in his twenties sitting slouched in a plastic chair. His eyes were heavy-lidded, as if he couldn't quite keep them open, and the care worker cupped her hand around the mug of tea he was trying to drink, to make sure it didn't fall.

She waved her hand for someone to take over helping the man, then stood up and came to us.

'Thank goodness you're here,' she said. 'We don't know what's going on.' She wrung her hands. 'Janice has gone to make him a sandwich. She won't be a minute.'

I looked at the man on the chair. He was dressed in an open-necked polo shirt covered in paint flecks and dust, and heavy-duty work trousers with Velcro pockets. Beside the stairs I could see a discarded tool belt with various-coloured handles tucked inside. Propped against the wall was a folded stepladder. I wondered whether he had fallen from the ladder.

'Hello there,' Ryan said, kneeling before the man. 'I've not met you before.'

The man's eyes were shut, his chin tucked down on his chest. He looked like he could fall off the chair at any minute.

'Hello, mate!' Ryan said more loudly, shaking the man's knee.

His eyes snapped open and then draped closed again, but he nodded his head as if he'd heard. He was responsive to voice.

'Can you tell me your name?' Ryan said.

The man opened his mouth; his lips were dry and stuck together.

'John,' he said, but the 'J' was sticky so that his name sounded more like 'Yohn'.

Ryan signalled to me to get the gear out.

'BP, ECG, blood sugar,' he said.

I unzipped the bag.

'Hello, John,' I said. 'I'm Molly. I'm just going to take some measurements from you, if that's okay.'

He nodded again and then yawned.

Janice came back with a sandwich on a floral china plate. She'd cut it into four neat triangles. Another care worker bit her nails nervously.

'We've got his mobile phone,' someone said. 'If it's helpful . . .' They trailed off. 'He's not been here long.'

I read out John's blood pressure and heart rate; both were stable and in range. I started attaching the ECG electrodes beneath his shirt. He didn't appear to notice.

'Okay then, John, how long have you been here at Brightside?'

John opened his eyes. He looked around him as if he couldn't remember being here at all. He swallowed slowly.

'He's not been here long, just fifteen minutes, and then this . . .'

Ryan looked back at the care worker biting her nails, his brow furrowed.

'What's his past medical history? Epilepsy?' he said, still crouched on the floor. 'Has he had a seizure?' He was loading up the blood glucose machine with a strip and rootling in the bag for a lancet to prick John's finger.

'We don't know!' The care worker threw her hands out. 'Like I said, he's not been here long. We don't know anything about him; we've not met him before!'

Ryan passed me the blood glucose monitoring kit.

'Okay, mate,' he said. 'Let's get you in the truck, and on the way we'll grab your notes from the front desk, have a read. Were you up that ladder?' He pointed.

John followed his finger. He nodded slowly.

'Lighhhh bulllb.' His voice was a drawl, like a paint-brush slopping fresh paint against the walls.

'Fixing the light bulbs,' Ryan repeated. 'Okay, I see. Good man.'

I cleaned John's index finger with cotton wool and water. It was warm, his palms clammy. His face was pale but his forehead was beaded with sweat. I explained that I was going to take a drop of blood from his finger.

Ryan knelt down beside me. 'A lot of the residents have jobs around the unit,' he told me. 'It's good for them, gives them some sense of the life they had before.'

He looked up at John, who was almost asleep.

'Take that sugar, Molly, and then let's get him in the truck.' He started to pack up.

John's head rolled, his eyes at half-mast.

'One point eight,' I said to Ryan.

He spun round.

'What?'

'One point eight,' I repeated.

Ryan looked at John.

'Repeat the test,' he said to me. He looked at the care workers hovering by the stairs. 'Is he a diabetic?' he asked them.

'We don't know!' Janice shouted. 'He's the handyman; he was called in to fix the upstairs lights.'

'One point eight,' I said. 'It definitely is.'

Low blood sugar, or hypoglycaemia, occurs when the level of glucose in the blood drops below 4.0 mmol/litre. The brain requires huge amounts of glucose to feed energy-demanding neurons, vital in maintaining brain function, and as a result, it is the body's main consumer of glucose. The brain has a protective permeable membrane called the blood–brain barrier, which places tight restrictions on what can and cannot pass through. Glucose is carried across this highly selective border with the aid of a transporter protein, a chaperone that safely diffuses it from the blood to the brain, allowing it to be used as energy. Brain signalling, computation and processing is reliant on this chemical exchange, and if glucose can't access the brain, a person will soon feel the debilitating effects.

People with diabetes have to monitor the sugar in their

blood more carefully than those who don't have the condition. Type 1 diabetics have a pancreas that does not produce insulin, the hormone needed to break down glucose from food. This means that they need to inject insulin themselves in order to keep the sugar level in their blood from being too high. Too much insulin or not enough food could send them into a hypoglycaemic state, and so it is important that the person checks their sugars regularly with a blood sugar monitoring kit. Type 2 diabetics might develop the condition later in life, whether it be for genetic reasons, lifestyle habits or diet. The pancreas is still able to produce insulin; however, it may not be enough, or the cells in the body might no longer respond to the release of the hormone. A person with type 2 diabetes may be able to manage their blood sugar levels by watching what they eat or drink; alternatively, they may need medication and some even use insulin injections.

The word 'diabetes' comes from the Greek *siphon*, and is credited to the physician Apollonius of Memphis, who noticed people suffering from a condition that produced excessive amounts of urine, their bodies siphoning off more fluid than they consumed. The word 'mellitus' was added later and derives from the Latin for 'honey', since it was noted (through bedside tasting) that the diabetic's urine tasted sweet, evidence of glucose in their waste product.

After the stomach operation I had to fix my swallowing problems as a teenager, I suffered from random episodes of severely low blood sugar. The first occurred ten years after my surgery, when I had completed my nurse training and was teaching a new overseas nurse on the cardiothoracic ward.

On shift, I became sweaty, my eyes unable to focus on the prescription chart during the medication round, and my mind felt far away. I presumed I had developed type 2 diabetes and decided to discuss the symptoms with a colleague's husband who was a type 1 diabetic and used to feeling the highs and lows of living with fluctuating blood sugar.

As we sat across from each other at the dinner table, he asked me if I remembered a Pot Noodle advert they showed many years ago on the TV. It featured a teenage boy sitting on the sofa about to open his heated-up instant snack. The camera zoomed in, showing the TV audience the red 'Extra Hot Chilli Fire' label on the outside of the container, engulfed by flames. The teenager took one mouthful and immediately exploded, his head blowing to pieces, his arms and legs and body shooting off in all directions so that all that was left on the sofa were the clothes he had been wearing, fixed in exactly the same position they had been in when his body inhabited them.

'It's like that,' my colleague's husband said, placing a single, pinpricked finger on the table to punctuate his point. 'When I saw that advert, the way his clothes are just left there, empty, I felt like that was the only way I could explain what low blood sugar feels like. As if you're far removed from where you've just been, but I couldn't tell you where.'

Back at Brightside Brain Injury Unit, Ryan unzipped the kit bag again and pulled out some GlucoBoost gel.

'Here, John, slurp this up. Where's that sandwich?' He reached across the carpet to pick it up. 'What's in it?'

'Jam!' someone shouted.

'Can you make us another tea?' I asked Janice. 'With lots of sugar.'

She scampered away.

'John, mate. Are you a diabetic?' Ryan asked.

John nodded. One arm slowly reached down to his pocket.

Ryan's gloved hand opened it for him and pulled out his insulin pen.

'Have you taken some?' Ryan said. John was too sleepy to answer. Ryan put a triangle of sandwich in his hand. 'Eat this.' He helped John bring the bread and jam to his mouth; John chewed at it slowly.

Janice brought more tea. John drank it.

The more he drank, the better his swallow and his grip became. He drank faster, chewed more purposefully, as if beginning to recognize his surroundings and the situation he found himself in.

'Recheck, Molly.'

I told John I was going to prick his finger.

'Two point five,' I said.

'Good,' Ryan said. 'Getting better. Keep eating, John. Then we'll get you in the truck and check you over.'

'Lucky I like jam sandwiches.' John's voice was clear this time, each word distinguishable from the last.

By the time he had finished the second sandwich, his blood sugar was 4.0 mmol/litre: stable. We let him rest back in the chair. He wiped his forehead and shivered.

'What happened, mate?' Ryan said, taking out his paperwork. 'Do you want to come and sit in the truck, or are you all right here?'

John looked about him.

'I'm okay,' he said. 'Thanks, ladies.' He grinned at the purple-garbed care workers leaning on the banister watching us. 'Well, I started at nine this morning but didn't have any calls lined up.'

'What do you do?' Ryan asked.

'Electrician,' John said. 'For some reason I was starving, so since I didn't have any jobs, I thought I'd get a McDonald's breakfast. I was in the drive-in queue and had the engine off. I'd already eyed up a big breakfast wrap with hash browns, so I gave myself a few units of insulin to cover it.'

Ryan nodded.

'Anyway, it was then that I got the emergency call from Brightside.' He gestured over to the carers. They nodded in agreement.

'It was urgent,' Janice said. 'All the lights had gone out; we couldn't see anything, couldn't help anyone out of bed, out of the bathroom . . .'

'It were dangerous,' someone else said.

'So I pulled out of the queue and made my way straight here. Completely forgot that I'd taken a shot of insulin just before and not bloody eaten anything to mop it all up. Next thing I know, I'm sitting on this chair with you feeding me a jam sandwich.'

'You don't remember anything before?' I asked.

John looked up to the ceiling. He wrinkled his nose.

'Not really. It's funny, actually.' He scratched his chin, able now to accurately place his hand there. 'Whenever I have a hypo, I feel like my mind has been somewhere else, but I can't for the life of me tell you where.' His eyes were fully open, the green irises speckled with yellow. 'Maybe there's some brain scan that can tell you where us diabetics drift off to.' He wiggled his fingers in front of him. 'Alien abduction?'

We all laughed.

John slapped his leg as if about to stand.

'Better give my missus a call,' he said.

'Do you feel better? Need to come with us to get checked over?'

John told us he would be fine now, that he would recheck his sugar as soon as he got back to his van and would eat another long-acting carbohydrate before he left. He shook both our hands and fixed the tool belt back around his waist.

'I'll get another leccy in to fix that last bulb,' he said to the care workers as he descended the stairs, throwing a hand up in goodbye.

They watched his every movement as he walked out of the door, gazing down at him from the landing as if he had just risen from the dead. Outside, the sky was as blue as it had been when we'd started our shift; the puffs of cloud had rolled away. There was nothing more to see here.

33

Despite advances in both brain imaging and space technology, the mysteries of consciousness and of dark matter remain unsolved. In outer space, dark matter is impossible to detect with current instruments and still remains a hypothesis, despite making up most of our universe. It consists of an invisible, exotic substance exerting a gravitational force on nearby objects; its existence is generally accepted due to its effect on galaxies, even though we are unable to see it. This is much like the workings of the mind. We know that memory exists; a healthy brain can recall memories at will and describe their intricacies clearly, but understanding how they are stored and retrieved is not so easily done.

This connection between our brains and outer space does not seem particularly surprising to nurses, who often comment that on a night with a full moon, the hospital sees more people suffering the effects of delirium. Delirium is common on the HDU, the elderly more likely to become acutely confused in the days after their operations.

From the Latin *de lira* (out of the furrow), delirium refers to a person no longer following their natural course, no longer tending to the soil in neat, ordered lines but rather deviating away towards a nonsensical path. This deviation in consciousness occurs without any evidence of its presence on CT scanners or in blood results to prove it existed at all.

In much the same way that dark matter causes a ray of light to stray from its natural path, the distortions that infiltrate our consciousness may be caused to ricochet to the forefront of our minds by some nebulous, undetectable brain matter lurking in the dark, droning universe that lies beneath our skull.

34

The next week, Dad was discharged home and I was back working on the HDU. I was looking after Shirley, a young woman suffering from an altered state of consciousness, her mind seeing things that couldn't be seen by others.

Shirley came from a town on the banks of the Thames estuary, bordered by marshes. She had collapsed at home; her sister, Charlie, had immediately started CPR, screaming at Shirley's two young children to run upstairs and call their Daddy; that Mummy had gone to sleep and auntie Charlie was helping her to wake up.

Charlie was the first-aider on site at the cleaning company she worked for, and had written notes during the training sessions to make sure she remembered it all. Later, she would describe to me how her hands were sweating when she stopped for a few seconds to call the ambulance. How her mobile had dropped to the floor, her slippery hands scrambling to hit speakerphone so that she could continue pounding her sister's chest with her interlaced fingers.

She could hear her niece and nephew crying upstairs, the little girl making the phone call to her daddy. She knew that Martin would be there in a matter of minutes, he worked on a construction site nearby.

She was out of breath by now. Shirley's lips were blue, her eyelashes were wet; Charlie wasn't sure if it was from her sweat or Shirley's tears. She stopped pumping Shirley's chest and bent down to breathe into her mouth, holding her nostrils closed with her fingers. The sweat was running down her neck, down the back of her shirt.

The ambulance crew were just round the corner, the faraway voice on the phone said. They told her to keep giving CPR; that the paramedics would be there to take over in under three minutes.

Martin crashed through the door. He clamped his hand over his mouth at the sight of his wife on the cold kitchen floor.

Charlie told him not to look, but to go upstairs to the kids. He disappeared at a run.

Charlie thought of the kids crying up there. She looked down at Shirley.

'Come on, Shirl,' she said.

Martin had left the front door open.

'Ambulance Service!' A shout came from the hallway.

Charlie kept pumping.

'She's here,' she said, but she could say no more; she was exhausted.

The two paramedics dropped to their knees beside Shirley. One of them unzipped the defibrillator whilst the other ripped open Shirley's T-shirt with his shears. They stuck the pads on her.

'Step back,' they said. 'We'll get her sorted; step back now.'

Martin came downstairs, his hand still clamped over his mouth. He stood and watched. Charlie stepped back beside him. Her hair was slicked to her forehead. 'Shockable rhythm,' the female paramedic said. They looked at the screen on the defibrillator, at the mad spidery black lines of Shirley's heart. 'Stand clear,' she instructed.

They took their hands off her.

Charlie looked away.

'Shock delivered,' the paramedic said.

They started pumping her chest again, still staring at the screen.

The female paramedic stood up and went to Martin. She put a hand on his arm.

'How long has she been like this?' She spoke quietly. Martin looked at his sister-in-law.

'Maybe three or four minutes before you arrived?' Charlie said.

'Has she got any problems with her heart that you are aware of?'

Martin shook his head.

She squeezed his arm, nodded and went back to her colleague on the floor.

Shock advised: the machine spoke.

'Stand clear,' the paramedic said, her eyes flitting from Shirley's body to the surrounding area, making sure everything was out of the way. 'Shock delivered.'

Shirley's chest bucked as if it had been struck by a bolt of lightning. Her whole body leapt from the floor.

Martin glanced away. She was looking less like Shirley now.

'Sinus rhythm.' The paramedic stopped pumping, took his hands from Shirley and stretched them out in front of him, clicking the joints in his fingers.

They tightened the oxygen mask around her face; her eyelashes started to flutter. They put a needle in her arm, took blood, drew up a crystal vial of something and gave it to her through her vein.

Martin went to his wife and held her hand. It was like ice. He turned it over in his own hand, searching for warmth.

'We've got her back,' the paramedic said. He put a hand on Martin's shoulder. 'You both did great, guys. You both did great.'

'Let's get her in,' the other paramedic said. 'I can hear HEMS outside.'

Charlie came and knelt beside Martin and her sister. They heard the vibration of the rotor blades. The helicopter was hovering, looking for a place to land. It scanned the marshes below, lit up silvery blue from the full moon hanging like a white lobe against the black sky.

Back at the hospital, I was starting a night shift. I finished my coffee, then went out to receive a bedside handover.

Shirley Mulligan, thirty-nine-year-old female, suffered an out-of-hospital cardiac arrest. Sister commenced CPR and once paramedics arrived two shocks were delivered. Return of spontaneous circulation. Air ambulance to King's and straight to cath lab, one stent placed in left circumflex. TR band removed from radial site, no bruising, no swelling, site has been intact since I've received her. Shirley has been stable post-procedure, observations as charted, apyrexial, sinus rhythm, maintaining good pressures. Post-op instructions are to continue on ACS protocol, cardiac monitoring and there's a CT head that they've just uploaded. I haven't had a chance to look yet . . .

I looked up from the chart to the nurse handing over.

She explained. 'Her GCS is fluctuating from thirteen to fourteen out of fifteen.'

This score on the Glasgow Coma Scale meant that Shirley had some degree of deficit in her consciousness. Whilst her eyes were open and she was able to obey movement-related commands, she was not orientated, she did not know where she was or what had happened to her, and questions she was asked became deflected and distorted in her mind.

I looked at her sitting upright talking to somebody on her phone, her husband's hand on her knee. She didn't look confused.

The nurse told me she wanted to show me the medication chart on the computers. I followed her to the nurses' station.

'I just wanted to say,' she said, her voice quiet, back turned to Shirley and her husband, 'she really *is* confused. She's been threatening to leave the ward and is quite aggressive, unfortunately.'

I nodded and thanked her.

Back at the bedside, I introduced myself. Martin told me the story of how Shirley's sister had started CPR and called the ambulance. He told me about what his kids had seen. Throughout the retelling of the story, Shirley clutched her mobile in her hand and stared at me through squinted eyes.

'Are you a prostitute?' she said. Her voice was calm and cut through the noise of the unit cleanly.

'Shirley,' I repeated, 'my name is Molly, I'm the nurse looking after you this evening.'

'Shirley, love, you're in the hospital . . . What's wrong with her?' Martin looked at me. 'Did the operation not go well?'

The cause of Shirley's cardiac arrest had been a blocked artery. In the cardiac cath lab they had inserted a small mesh tube into one of the arteries supplying her heart to keep the vessel open. The operation had gone well.

Cardiac arrest is attributed to an electrical malfunction within the heart. The heart starts to beat chaotically without a synchronized rhythm and is unable to work effectively as a pump. The blockage in Shirley's artery had disturbed the flow of blood to her heart muscle, a heart attack, leading it to beat abnormally as a response: a cardiac arrest. This abnormal heart rhythm became dangerous; the organ was no longer able to pump blood and oxygen around her body, so Shirley stopped breathing and became unconscious.

'Didn't know you liked prozzies,' she said, and started getting out of the chair, tugging on her urinary catheter as if it was anchoring her there, and unclipping the cardiac leads from her chest.

'What the fuck are you doing, Shirley? Have you lost your mind?'

'Piss off,' Shirley said.

'Your family saved your bloody life!' Martin said. 'And this is the thanks we're gonna get!'

'Saved my life? Ruined it, don't you think? Things haven't been the same since . . .'

Martin looked at me, confused, his hands outstretched. 'What's going on?' he said. 'Have you given her something to make her like this? Shirley, what are you talking about?'

'Maybe if you could step out for a minute,' I said to him, 'me and Shirley can get sorted.'

'Slut,' she said to me as he left.

I sat down on a footstool. Shirley was barely five foot tall and must have weighed about seven stone. She had thin light-blonde hair tied back in a ponytail, and was wearing joggers and a sparkly T-shirt that was on back to front. She must have tried to dress herself after coming out of the cath lab. The catheter hung awkwardly over the waistband of her joggers. I wanted to fix it in case it caused her injury, but knew she wouldn't allow me to touch her.

'Tell me how you're feeling,' I said. All the curtains were pulled around us. I could hear my colleagues wheeling the drug trolleys down the unit, starting their medication round, checking the wall oxygen, the emergency bags, the suction, the crash bells. Getting ready for the night.

'Like you care,' she said, and began packing her rucksack. She stuffed in toilet paper, the hospital menu, a patient gown that was draped across the bed.

'Listen,' I said. 'Shirley, you're here at the hospital because you had a heart attack at home.'

She ignored me.

'Because you were on the floor without oxygen for quite a bit of time, your brain has become muddled up. We need to look after you in here whilst it gets better.'

She twisted her mouth to the side, pursing her lips.

'He tried to kill me,' she said.

I listened.

'Probably wanted me dead this time and all. Things haven't been the same since they died.'

'I think your husband was there when they were doing CPR,' I said quietly. 'I'm sure that was very upsetting for him.'

She tutted loudly and continued packing.

'Do you think you could stay here just for tonight?' I tried.

'Get Martin,' she barked at me.

I brought Martin back in; he smelt of cigarette smoke and night air.

'What's going on, love?' he said to Shirley. He sat down on the bed watching her cramming items into the rucksack. 'You can't come home; you've gotta get checked over. You nearly died tonight.'

'That's what *she* said. You've been talking to her.'

'She's the nurse!' he said. 'Of course I'm bloody talking to her.'

I went out to find the nurse in charge. Time was moving and I still had another patient to look after. I had been warned during handover that Shirley was confused, but it seemed as if she might be a higher risk than that and might even try to leave the unit. I thought we should probably let security know.

After that, I loaded her CT scan up on the computer to take a better look. Shirley's round glowing head appeared before me like a map of the night sky. I could see the white rim of her skull encasing a mass of grey fissures and cisterns, shadowy canals and sinuses that led to more darkness, half-lit lobes and inky ventricles that looked pitch black and starless.

Thankfully the scan didn't reveal any great changes to

Shirley's brain, though the radiographer had noted that it was swollen, the grey looking murkier in some areas due to an accumulation of fluid. The doctors would re-scan her in the coming days to see if the darkness enveloping it had reduced. According to the notes attached to the images, the swelling was most likely a result of the hypoxic brain injury sustained when her brain had not received enough oxygen during resuscitation. Shirley was suffering the effects of reperfusion, a condition in which blood flow has returned to the brain and a subsequent overwhelming inflammatory response is initiated, causing brain dysfunction.

The aim of cardiopulmonary resuscitation (CPR) is to take over the function of the heart whilst it is no longer working, propelling blood to the brain using the pumping action of the hands to preserve brain function. By initiating CPR, Charlie had saved her life.

Mouth-to-mouth resuscitation was first recommended for drowning victims in the mid eighteenth century. Amsterdam, with its winding canals and high incidence of drowning, founded a society for 'Resuscitating the Drowned' and promoted the mouth-to-mouth technique to restore life. Other methods aiming to bring people back from near-death had previously been used with little success; they included suspending a person by the heels to promote air flow, and rectal fumigation – using tobacco smoke blown up the rectum to stimulate the heart to beat and the person to breathe. Fumigators and bellows were hung along the Thames in case a passer-by came across an apparently dead person and might be able to use the equipment to save them.

In the first book of Kings in the Old Testament of the Bible, the prophet Elisha laid himself on a lifeless child, placing his eyes against the child's eyes, his hands against his hands and his mouth against his mouth until the flesh of the child became warm again. Medical journals and textbooks have recognized this biblical passage as an early example of mouth-to-mouth resuscitation. Before this, the ancient Egyptian winged goddess Isis breathed life into her newly dead husband so that they could conceive a son together before he descended into the Underworld to rule. Osiris's resuscitation was temporary, and it is believed in some Egyptian mythology that Isis's tears of mourning for her husband caused the flooding of the Nile each year.

Hypoxic brain injury occurs when oxygen supply is interrupted. This interruption can be from heart attack, cardiac arrest or non-cardiac-related events such as drowning, choking, asthma attack or even climbing to high altitudes. Travellers along the ancient Silk Road named a particular stretch of peaks Great Headache Mountain and Little Headache Mountain to describe the effects of climbing to extreme heights where the air was thin and there was little oxygen. Vomiting, confusion and hallucinations were reported, and in the late twentieth century, British mountaineers and doctors together began to look into ways to remedy the effects of high altitude.

With decreased blood flow and little oxygen, Shirley's brain had been forced to try and function with a depleted energy source. As a result, its electrical charge and its production of the neurotransmitters that had been helping to send clear messages throughout her body had been altered. Shirley's brain was now a constellation of molecular black-outs, burnt-out stars and pockets of vacuum-like space.

On the outside, she looked like Shirley, but her sense of herself no longer seemed to be confined to its borders. She had little recollection of the days leading up to her heart attack, as her short-term memory had been almost completely erased. Her image of herself, which was once defined and determinable, was now warped, her thoughts bowed outwards as if her waterlogged brain exerted extra pressure on its foundations. She was irritable, disorientated and suspicious of everything around her.

'How long do I have to stay?' She turned around to face me.

'Shirley, love,' Martin pleaded with her. 'You've had a heart attack. You've got to stay until they've checked you're all right.'

'I haven't had a heart attack.' She showed her teeth. 'You're all trying to keep me here. You're gonna take the kids.'

Martin raised his arms and let them drop to his sides. He exhaled noisily and pushed the curtain aside to leave. Out on the unit, I could see my other patient, an elderly woman who was not long out of theatre, sleeping peacefully beside the nurses' station.

'Who's that?' Shirley snapped at me. She had seen me looking beyond the curtain.

'It's another patient, Shirley. We've got nine other patients here tonight and we really want you to stay so we can look after you too.'

'Fine,' she said, and sat down on the bed. She pulled the blankets up around her, folded the top of the sheet down over her eyes.

Quietly I drew the curtains back so that we could see her.

The nurse in charge caught my eye. I nodded. We had made it through the first hour.

Martin left around midnight. The night was long. Every time I went to record Shirley's observations, she would wake and try and get out of bed. Each time I managed to persuade her to stay, just an hour longer, just for the night, until she fell into a deep sleep at about three in the morning.

There is a feeling one gets at three or four in the morning on a night shift, just as night is slipping into day. It's a sliding sensation, as if you are lying flat and being pushed head first down a slope, the blood rushing to your head, pressure building behind the eyes. It's as if both ears are blocked with water and everything you do, from picking up a cup to running your hands under a tap, is happening very far away. It's not you, but you watching yourself, a tiny speck of glitter and dust orbiting the HDU far off in the distance. Nobody ever mentioned this feeling during my nurse training. Now I watched myself watching Shirley sleep.

A couple of hours later, she was woken by her own visions. She jumped out of bed and pointed at the corner of the room, her finger unwavering in the dark.

I went to her but was careful not to touch her.

'It's okay,' I said.

'Look,' she said, and stretched her arm as long and

straight as she could to the window frame on the other side of the unit, where the moon shone through. 'It's them.'

The other nurses glanced up from the station, their faces illuminated by phone and computer screens. Shirley was whispering loudly, her eyes round, pupils dilated, taking in the night.

'Shirley, remember you're with us at the hospital. You need to rest.'

She didn't hear me; her finger was a long, straight antenna scanning the blackness.

'They're right there,' she said. 'Two girls and a boy.'

Her eyes didn't move. I followed her gaze but saw only the moon in the window pane, the sleeping patient beneath with a bag of fluid quietly dripping into her veins.

'The ones I lost,' she whispered. 'My babies . . .'

The nurse in charge came over. We looked at each other. We let Shirley talk, her voice a hoarse whisper. She put a hand over her mouth as if to quieten herself. Her eyes were wide.

'And so gorgeous,' she sighed. 'Just like I knew they would have been.'

She looked at me to see if I agreed. I nodded and smiled.

'Those beautiful halos,' she said. 'Like little stars above their heads. The ones I lost, those babies that were never really gone.' She waved into the darkness, her hand splayed as if against glass. It was the first time I had seen her smile. 'Look at them!' she said. 'Standing in a row, waiting for me! My bright little stars . . .'

Gently the nurse in charge put her hand on the small of Shirley's back and led her to her bed. She didn't resist.

I tucked her in and reattached the cardiac leads to her chest without saying a thing. Shirley was still smiling, staring with unblinking eyes at the patch of darkness where she had seen the children, her babies, the ones she had lost, waiting for her beneath the hospital's celestial colonnades.

In the morning, she didn't remember her hallucinations. She sipped sweet tea from a blue beaker and scrolled through her phone, unaware that her thoughts had veered off course overnight. She was calmer and I was able to take her observations without upsetting her. Her blood pressure and heart rate were stable; it was only her brain that was still recovering from the heart attack. The doctors would re-scan her today and she would be seen by the hypoxic brain injury team and the occupational therapists.

I got a coffee for the way home, and as I drove, I listened to the news on the radio. It talked of a meteor shower forecast to occur that night.

35

Shirley would make a full recovery, although she would probably never remember the cardiac arrest or much about her stay in hospital. Others who have taken longer to resuscitate have a more uncertain recovery, their brains appearing in scans much darker than they once were.

A vegetative state is a disorder of consciousness that can develop after a brain injury. A person who has suffered a cardiac arrest with a significant downtime (the time on the ground being resuscitated) may appear in a vegetative state, a state of wakefulness but without any awareness of their surroundings. Their eyes may be open but they lack any purposeful movements, language or comprehension and are unable to express themselves in any form. They may have a breathing tube, be unable to eat and drink for themselves, and be incontinent. Whilst they may open and close their eyes in patterns that imitate sleep, their sleep/wake cycle, which is controlled by the brain, has been disturbed and often their eyes will be open in the middle of the night and closed when the most stimulating, noisy family members have come to visit.

Prognosis is difficult and depends on a variety of factors, including cause of hypoxia, age, length of downtime, degree and location of damage to the brain.

*

Ranjit was from the north of India, a desert city called Jais-almer, strewn with sandstone havelis with ornate balconies and internal courtyards sparkling with coloured-glass lanterns. I had visited the sand city with Rob on a trip to India years earlier.

In India, Ranjit had worked as a lecturer and had a son and a daughter with his wife. They had moved to the UK when the children were still young. He had been working from home when he suffered a heart attack. His wife believed he had been on the floor for at least twenty minutes, as they had spoken on the phone as she was driving home, and when she got to the house she had found him collapsed. She called an ambulance and they arrived within five minutes and began CPR. The paramedics gave him three shocks and were able to restart his heart. He was blue-lighted to hospital and remained in an induced coma in intensive care for two weeks. It was unclear how his brain would recover when he was weaned from the infusions keeping him asleep.

When he came out of the coma, he was moved to the HDU, since he no longer required the use of a ventilator and was able to breathe for himself. His wife waited outside whilst we transferred him over to our monitors and pumps and made sure he was settled. We put the brakes on the bed and the intensive care nurse disconnected her portable monitor whilst I attached our cardiac leads to Ranjit's chest. I leant over him and noticed that his cheeks were streaked with wet, as if he had been crying. The intensive care nurse had put paraffin on his lips to heal the cracks and his hair was slicked down to one side with water. She tidied his belongings away in his new locker: sponge bag, short-sleeved shirt, trousers and leather belt, clothes that he hadn't worn for weeks. She tucked his shoes at the bottom of the locker, the laces tied neatly in little bows like kisses. I wondered if his wife had done that or if his shoes had remained untouched since the last time he stepped out of them.

I said hello to Ranjit and squeezed his hand. I told him my name and that I would be looking after him; that he had been stepped down from intensive care and that he was doing well. He didn't open his eyes; his teeth ground in his mouth, creaking back and forth like a rusty swing after dark.

When we finished the handover, I reattached his bag of feed, a creamy brown liquid full of vitamins and electrolytes that drip-fed through a tube in his nose down into his stomach. Sometimes he would lick his lips or twist his tongue in his mouth, but these seemed to be reflexive movements; he was not aware he was doing them. When his eyes did open, they roved the room like spinning planets but never came to rest on anything or anyone in front of him. When he yawned, I would get a chance to see whether I could clean his mouth, softly scraping his tongue or running a mouthwash sponge over his teeth. At times the task would make him clamp down on the sponge and I would try to get him to relax his jaw, stroking both his arms, running my fingers up towards his cheeks until he loosened his grip.

His wife came in and stood beside him, taking his hand in hers. She unfurled his tightly clenched fingers and let them rest in her palm. She spoke to him gently in Hindi and rubbed the back of his hand with her thumb.

Ranjit had a tracheostomy in his throat that he breathed through. He didn't require oxygen any more but we put a little filter on the end of the tube to warm and humidify the air he was taking in. His chest sounded wet, and when he inhaled and exhaled you could hear the sticky secretions gurgling in his lungs. I asked his wife if she could give us five minutes to sit him up more comfortably to help him breathe.

She nodded and once again waited outside behind the swing doors.

We worked quickly. I turned off the feed so that he wouldn't accidentally breathe it into his lungs whilst he was lying down flat. We lowered the bed, reassuring him that we would have him sitting up soon. The healthcare assistant and I took turns to hold him close to us whilst we rolled him, checking his skin was soft and smooth and not yet damaged by days spent lying in bed. We rubbed cream on his back and the creases of his bottom, then put pillows beneath the sheet on one side to take the pressure off the area. We fixed the catheter tubing to his leg and made sure it wasn't kinked and was still draining into the bag.

When we sat him up in the bed, I reapplied the oxygen probe and could hear and see that he needed to have the secretions in his chest cleared. I placed an oxygen mask over his breathing tube that nebulized salty water into a fine mist to help loosen anything that needed to come up. Using sterile gloves, I passed a thin sterile tube attached to suction down his tracheostomy to just before a ridge of cartilage in his chest where the trachea divided into right and left bronchi. This stimulated his cough and he was able to shift some of the wetness for himself. I held the tube firmly and withdrew it, managing to clear creamy white secretions that had been causing the problem. Afterwards I applied a nebulizer filled with more saline water to loosen the remainder of the secretions and made sure Ranjit could rest from the procedure.

His wife came back in and we talked about their family. Ranjit and Deepa had been married for forty years and were hoping to travel back to Rajasthan with the children the following year to celebrate their ruby anniversary; he had bought her the stone already. She told me she worried her children would forget the place they were born, and she wanted to stay in India for a month or two so that they could spend time with all the family. Her son worked for Transport for London now and her daughter was in her final year of teacher training.

'For us, education is everything,' she said. 'We wanted to give our children the best chance at pursuing their studies, and when an opportunity came up for Ranjit in England, we knew we had to go. We wanted to go!' She laughed. 'I'll never forget the look on Ranjit's face when we made the decision.' She looked at him as if hoping to see the expression again now. 'He was so excited,' she sighed. 'Well . . .' She paused. 'I'm grateful we're here now. You nurses . . .' She smiled and held her hands out, palms upturned, as if reading the lines across them but not being able to see where they ended up.

I told her I had been to India many times; that my parents had taken me there as a child and that I had taken Rob years later when we went backpacking round the world after university. I told her that my dad had gone to India for the first time over thirty years ago. After his trip, Dad knew he wanted to take his own family there one day. India had become like a story passed down through our family.

In the years before my sister and I were born, Dad travelled to India to cover a jazz festival for the music newspaper *Melody Maker*. The Jazz Yatra took place in a park in Mumbai (then Bombay) and saw musicians from all over the world make the long trip. The Charlie Mingus memorial band had never been to India before, but Mingus's widow had flown out just the year before to scatter his ashes in the Ganges River. She was back this year to hear the band play his music. It was February. Dad left Mum and a rainy London and boarded his flight. As they came in to land, the pilot told them over the Tannoy not to be alarmed if they looked out of the window and saw the whole city suddenly go dark. India was about to experience a total solar eclipse.

'I remember that eclipse!' Deepa laughed, one hand resting on the bed. 'Ranjit had been talking about it for weeks before. We took the train to the Jantar Mantar in Jaipur to see it, you know; have you been there?'

The Jantar Mantar is the world's largest sundial. Its looming slopes were built in the eighteenth century. Mum and Dad had taken us to see it when we were children. We travelled across the north of the country by car and I vividly remember the space towers and celestial cupolas scraping the sky. The universe was so close. It felt as if you could stretch a hand out and feel the clink of stars like loose change caught between your fingers.

'Back then,' she said, 'you could climb all over them, before they were cordoned off. Ranjit was like a child that day.' She looked at her husband and smiled. 'I can see him now, running ahead of Chandra and Mihir, leaping up the steps of the eclipse tower two at a time until he got to the highest point. It was only when he reached the top that he looked back and remembered us all waiting at the bottom! He took Chandra's hand and made sure she was right at the front, right up high, you know. He wanted her to see it perfectly up there.'

Deepa straightened Ranjit's sheet, her face bowed to the bed.

That afternoon I looked at Ranjit's brain scan on the computer. There was wide-ranging damage to various areas of his brain, including the frontal lobe, where high cognitive functions such as memory and problem-solving exist. The notes attached to the scan detailed that his brain injury was diffuse, the swelling spread out over a large area.

Over the next month, his condition did not change, and the doctors now described him as being in a continuing vegetative state. He still lacked any awareness of himself or his surroundings, and any action he did make seemed entirely automatic.

During the ward round, Deepa asked when he would

be able to squeeze her hand. The team found it hard to offer a prognosis. The likelihood of significant cognitive improvement would decrease as the days went on, but it was still too early to be completely certain. In the UK, it is suggested that brain injuries such as Ranjit's may be judged permanent if there are no signs of improvement after six months.

At the end of the week, he had an EEG, which recorded and measured electrical activity in his brain through sticky probes attached to the scalp. The EEG is used to offer a window into the brain's inner workings, transcribing electrical patterns onto the screen to reveal how it is functioning in the form of brain waves. These waves swing back and forth at different speeds and amplitudes depending on the state of the patient. Brains that are alert and thinking might reveal a predominance of beta waves, fast-paced, lurching forward to the next peak, conveying engagement and high levels of arousal.

Ranjit's brain scan revealed mainly delta and theta waves, slow-brain activity resembling deep sleep or the state just before falling asleep. In the low light of the scanner, his eyes were closed; the landscape of his brain was dark.

Suddenly, something flickered across the screen, streaks of light cast against the dark dome of his skull. His brain was exhibiting cortical responses, sparking on either side like tiny fires in the distance. The technician leant in closer, examining the brain waves, the hypnotic breakers crashing against the grey shores of Ranjit's frontal lobe. The deep mountain ranges of his brain waves were vast and yawning, delta waves producing a pure sonorous vibration, not words or sound, but tremors that boomed across his cortex, deafening and yet unheard inside his skull.

When we wheeled him back to the unit, his eyes were open. We hoisted him into his tilted chair and supported his arms, legs and head with pillows. Deepa came to visit and sat beside him holding his hand.

'How has he been?' she asked me.

'All his observations are good,' I said. 'He's had his eyes closed for much of the day.'

'You need to wake up, Ranjit. You've done enough sleeping now.' She rubbed his hand and rested her chin on her own hand, watching him. There were dark smudges beneath her eyes.

'How are you doing?' I asked her.

'I'm fine,' she said quietly. 'I have to be.' She looked at me. 'He has to know I am okay out here so that he can focus on getting himself better in there. See, Ranjit, I'm fine out here.'

'He had his scan today,' I said. 'The electrical scan of his brain. I'm just waiting for the report to be uploaded.'

'Was there any electricity?' She looked up at me.

'Yes,' I said. 'There was brain activity.'

'I feel like it must be so dark in there.' She rubbed her own head. 'Like an eclipse!' She smiled at me. 'And we're just waiting for the light to come back.' She started to cry.

'I'm sorry,' I said. I held her tightly and felt her shuddering; the tears didn't stop. 'You're doing so well. I can't imagine how hard this is.'

'Oh goodness,' she said at last, exhausted from crying.

She turned back to Ranjit, smiling once again. His eyes were open, fixed and staring at the closed curtain ahead.

'Ranjit, darling,' she said, and held his face in her hands.

'Chandra is going to be a teacher. She has been awarded a first-class degree at university.'

Ranjit closed his eyes. A single tear fell.

'Don't you cry.' Deepa wiped it away with her thumb. 'Don't you cry now.'

Ranjit opened his mouth.

'Chandra,' he whispered.

He had spoken. One single sound had slipped from his lips; glittering with gold, it hung in the air like a decoration. His daughter's name sounded like the first sound the world made, bright as the first flare peeping out from behind the eclipse.

Exposure

The wound is the place where the light enters you.

Rumi

36

We were in France. Dad was back in the water. It was warm and sun-touched on the surface, but cool as stone below where our toes nestled in the shingle. There were pine needles drifting lazily past on the top of the lake, and my sister's little girl, Dotty, rode an inflatable turtle in the shallows. Dad stood with the water up to his waist. His long heart surgery scar was pink and white in the sunlight but well healed.

I watched them both, Dad wading and Dotty floating. When I was Dotty's age, I had a teddy bear that unzipped at the back; a long silver scar that opened down to its middle. You could reach inside and feel the bear's stuffing and its soft silk lining, but if you dug a little deeper, you could feel its heart; you could lock your fingers around it and feel it beating.

I floated on my back, one hand across my stomach. I could feel my own scars there, five keyhole slits, now white and raised since the years had passed and scar tissue had formed, distinguished by its thick fibrous architecture. After my stomach surgery, the skin had rebuilt harder, forming around the injury as if remembering the trauma and barricading itself against the next.

The word 'scar' derives from fourteenth-century Old French, *escharre*, which in turn comes from the Latin *eschara* and the Greek *eskhara*, 'a scab forming in response to a burn'; literally 'a hearth or fireplace'.

The make-up of scar tissue is vastly different to that of normal skin. After an injury, the body bleeds and quickly forms a clot that hardens into a protective scab to stem the flow. From here a glue-like protein called collagen is produced and lies across the wound in straight ordered lines parallel to the rest of the skin. This is entirely different to normal, uninjured skin, which forms in a random cross-weave structure like thousands of miniature diamonds strewn across the surface in no particular order.

In French, there are phrases originating far back in the seventeenth century and still used today: *se faire la peau de quelqu'un*, meaning to kill someone but directly translated as 'to have one's skin', or *risquer sa peau*, 'to risk one's skin', as if the skin of the person represents them as a whole.

Out of the water and under the shade of the pines we gathered on the hard-packed earth. We had travelled to France for family holidays since I was a child, since Verdon Gorge and the day my dad's hand pulled me out from the fast-flowing river.

We reapplied suntan lotion and ate a lunch of bread and cheese, sliced apples and plump tomatoes, the juice dribbling down Dotty's little fingers. She laughed. My sister rocked baby Mabel to sleep. Daisy's husband and Rob kicked a ball around near the lake. The air was filled with laughter, people splashing, falling off rubber rings, screeching and screaming. A woman and her young daughter walked by, both wrapped in towels, clutching melting ice creams and bags of steaming chips, the paper translucent with grease and twinkling salt streaks.

Dad sat on a low camping chair propped up against a tall tree. Once he had finished lunch, he rested his head back against the gnarled bark and pulled his white panama hat over his eyes to sleep. He had worn that hat on every childhood holiday I could remember.

Dotty rushed back into the water with Mum whilst Daisy and I watched. They crashed through the shallows, knees up high until they could run no more, and fell, tumbling and laughing together, into the lake.

When we got back to the campsite, Dad rested on the bed. He was getting tired more easily since the operation, but the surgeons had assured us that it was normal, that his body was still carrying a lot of excess fluid that would tire him out before it drained. His leg was swollen where they had taken the vein and used it in his heart. The more he moved around and stayed active, the more quickly the swelling would start to diminish. But that afternoon, he slept on top of the thin cotton covers in the waning heat of the day.

We walked to the campsite pool down a dusty path. There were slides and waterfalls, and a wooden hut playing loud summertime music from shuddering speakers. Dotty squeezed her armbands back on, the plastic still warm from lying in the sun by the lake. Daisy and her husband and Rob and I found some loungers and stretched out to read our books whilst Mum took Dotty into the busy pool. We saw them and then we didn't; no doubt the two of them had ducked beneath a waterfall, or were exploring the waterslides and the lazy river. I lay back on the lounger and stared up at the unwavering dark green pines against the pure blue of the sky.

Dad arrived an hour or so later. He had a small canvas bag slung over one shoulder, his glasses and a book inside. His panama hat was creased at the brim where it had been squashed in the car on the way back from the lake.

We waved and he saw us. I pulled a plastic chair over and he put his bag beside it. He leant on the railing and stared out at the beach below, the rocky cliff face upon which the swimming pool and the campsite rested. From this distance the beach was yellow and the water had just a few waves cresting; the heat made everything very still. Dad looked directly down, peering over the railing to see the sheer face, the rocky ridge, the fallen pine needles, the dust and scuttling beetles with their oil-spill shells.

'Dad,' I said. He was leaning too far over the railing.

He turned his face towards me and his panama hat fell from his head. We all stood quickly and watched it fall, bumping over stones and shells and sandstone and dust, gathering speed and picking up pine needles in its brim until it came to a stop, wedged between a twisted root and a rock.

'Dad!' I said again. 'Your hat . . .'

He touched his hand to his head as if trying to hold the memory of the panama in place.

Mum and Dotty came out of the water; Dotty's little cheeks were pink and she panted as she half skipped towards us.

'What are you looking at?' Mum asked, seeing us all assembled beside the railing.

'Dad's hat,' I said, and pointed.

Mum came to look. Dotty peered through the metal railings.

'Bobo's hat!' She looked up at her grandfather. 'What do we do?'

'I'm going to get it,' I said.

Rob and I peered down the steep drop.

'You are not,' my mum said.

'Don't worry about it, Mol,' Dad said. 'I've got plenty more at home.'

'Not this hat,' I said. 'You've had this one for years.'

We all looked down at it again, perfectly white, pricked with pine needles.

'I'll go,' Rob said. He had flip-flops and swimming trunks on.

'Nobody's going,' Mum said. 'It'll just have to stay there.'

'What, forever?' Dotty said, pressing her face closer to the railings.

'As long as it lasts,' Mum said.

'It was a good weave, that hat.' Dad took his eyes from it. 'Intricate. Three thousand weaves per square inch, they told me.'

'It was your hat,' I said plainly.

We all turned away from the hat on the cliff face and went back to reading our books on the loungers. Dad moved further into the shade to keep the worst of the sunshine from his skin. I didn't want to read; I stared up at the blue and green again, a clew suspended in the expanse.

I thought about Dad's hat. I wondered whether it would

change with the seasons, or the tide, or the salinity of the ocean, the rocks eroding, the earth contracting and expanding as time passed. I thought, if we ever came back to this campsite, years in the future, and climbed down to fetch the hat from between the rock and the twisted root, we would see that the weave had changed, just as skin changes after an injury, after time has passed without us there. I wondered if we might see that the straw was no longer cross-weaved as Dad had known it, but now formed of straight bands, all facing one direction like scar tissue, regrouping after the trauma of being left behind.

37

In the Resuscitation Council's guidelines on conducting an ABCDE assessment, the section relating to exposure – the examination of the skin and the body as a whole – comprises just two sentences. Breathing consists of twelve paragraphs, circulation nineteen. But looking at the body as a whole is fundamental to understanding a patient's condition. The wounds and scars they have acquired through their life help us understand a person's story, the world they live in, where they have come from, what they have endured.

The nurse must look at a patient from head to toe, exposing them fully whilst both maintaining their dignity and minimizing heat loss. Through the skin we might find the source of their condition: low blood pressure from a haemorrhaging wound uncovered beneath a T-shirt, pain from a fractured femur pushing against a trouser leg, a rash signalling an allergic reaction spreading out across the back.

Whilst E is the fifth part of the nursing assessment, representing the final stage, it does not represent the end. The A–E examination is fluid and can move backwards as well as forwards. Upon reaching the fifth part of the examination, one might be led back to the start: what if this mark on the person's skin is the cause of their neurological condition in D; what if their neurological condition is the cause of their breathing problem in B? What if, what if . . .

During the first four parts of the assessment, the nurse has predominantly focused on the inside of the body, shining pen torches within the mouth to look for possible obstructions blocking the airway; listening to the inside of the chest, to damaged lungs or creaky heart valves; staring into the dark depths of brain scans searching for the origins of consciousness inside the skull.

Exposure, in contrast, offers an opportunity to focus on the outside, to look for elements of the self on the surface. For thousands of years the skin was interpreted in this way, perceived as a porous surface that offered clues as to what was happening on the inside. This approach to the outer layer of the body would begin to wane with the evolution of clinical-anatomical medicine in the eighteenth century.

Before this evolution, if there were no natural opening in the body, the physician would make one in order to allow the sickness to pass; blood-letting, scarification and acupuncture were common practices to try and alleviate the symptoms of disease via the skin.

Whilst the study of anatomy through dissection has a long history, dating as far back as ancient Greece, it wasn't until Flemish anatomist Andreas Vesalius's pioneering work with dissection in the sixteenth century that pre-established thinking was revolutionized. Prior to him, the world generally accepted the anatomical writings and dogmatic teachings of Galen, much of which was based on dissection of animals rather than human beings.

With the coming of the Enlightenment period, the practice of dissecting cadavers was widespread across medical schools and in anatomical theatres (when corpses were available). The new, modern body was no longer interpreted purely by changes on its surface, nor was it so widely thought to be connected to the external world by osmotic, visceral projections such as blood and urine. Instead it had come to be understood as a demarcated boundary, a passage into an internal realm that could be scientifically and objectively explored through the physician's skill.

The first time I saw *inside* was as a teenager. In the years before my stomach surgery, we went to Professor Gunther von Hagens' exhibition 'Body Worlds' in east London. This exhibition hosted twenty-five cadavers, stripped bare of their skin, flayed, bisected and dissected, and safely ensconced in revolving glass cases. These dead bodies had been through an innovative process called plastination, in which the cells of the body were impregnated with liquid polymer in order to preserve the cadaver for viewing.

The image of one body in particular stayed with me. I remember looking up at the corpse suspended behind glass; pink and red and taut with stretched sinew and ligaments. This écorché stood upright with one foot in front of the other, head tilted, looking glassily at its own skin, which hung lifelessly from its outstretched arm like a wet raincoat, collapsed and empty of its body. Later I learnt that it was based on a famous sixteenth-century copperplate illustration of a flayed cadaver holding its own skin aloft, the dagger used in the flaying held in the other hand. In the illustration, the face left behind in the discarded skin looked haunted, nothing more than five black holes for eyes, nose and a mouth, perhaps the last expression it wore before it was skinned alive.

When we returned home from the exhibition, I stood in front of the mirror and examined my own skin. I could hardly believe that a von Hagens-type structure lived beneath. My own skin was smooth; it had lived for fifteen years and not yet picked up any scars or wrinkles. I had my mum's delicate hands and my dad's round fingernails.

One year later, I stood in the same spot and examined my skin once again. I had come home from the hospital in springtime, the tree outside Daisy's bedroom pink with blossom. Mum helped me walk to the front door on a carpet of petals.

Over the next few weeks, I stood in front of the mirror and watched my stomach scars heal. One of the scars took longer than the others; it itched through the night and when I looked at it closely it appeared more open than the others. It seemed as if I was staring into something elemental, some blood-red part of me that had always been there but that I had not seen before. This new layer seemed both concealing and revealing at the same time.

38

Wound care has been in existence for thousands of years. Some of its most fundamental steps have been practised since ancient times. Egyptians used honey to protect wounds from infection and adhesive dressings to keep them dry, whilst the ancient Greeks recognized the signs of infection and the value of cleanliness, which is at the heart of contemporary medical practice.

Some wounds require vacuum-assisted therapy to draw bacteria out from the inside in order to help them close and heal. This practice of sucking out excess fluid, clots and bacteria is a technique that has been employed as far back as the Trojan War.

A modern-day Greek professor of medicine and his colleagues conducted a review of the injuries sustained within Homer's *Iliad*. They ranked arrow wounds at a 42 per cent mortality rate, slingshot wounds at 67 per cent and sword wounds at a devastating 100 per cent. The harsh realities of the battlefield, in particular the chaotic close combat experienced during the Trojan War, meant that many soldiers sustained deep, penetrating open wounds that could quickly develop infection in the basic environment.

In his epic poem, Homer describes how brave King Menelaus of Sparta is injured by an arrow. A nearby physician quickly tends to him, pulling out the arrow and sucking forth the blood from the wound before applying a dressing. This negative-pressure technique was similarly used by the Roman army, which employed specialist wound-suckers on the battlefield to place their mouths around a soldier's wound in order to draw out foreign objects, poisons or blood and allow the injury to heal.

The practice of wound-sucking developed into glass cupping, which also provided a vacuum seal for drainage. This vacuum-assisted method continued into the eighteenth century, when noblemen would ask for a type of wound-sucker to be brought to them when they were challenged to a duel.

Florence Nightingale realized during the Crimean War that soldiers were predominantly dying from unsanitary conditions rather than the severity of their wounds. Her pioneering notes on nursing still inform our work more than one hundred and fifty years later.

I was taught how to apply negative-pressure wound therapy in my first year as a nurse on the vascular ward. The modern-day method comes in the form of an electronic box attached to a drainage tube, and is applied using a flexible sponge and transparent dressing to form a vacuum seal over the wound. The patient can walk around with the drainage box neatly hung from a strap over their shoulder. The nurse looking after the patient will monitor both the vacuum for battery life and its dressing to ensure a good seal is maintained. Once the box is turned on, the pressure is set to − 125 mm of mercury to draw out excess fluid, blood and bacteria whilst simultaneously promoting blood flow to the area in order to help its edges come together.

I learnt quickly about the art of negative-pressure wound therapy, the skill of securely cutting and shaping the sponge to the exact contours of a person's skin to ensure the seal is tight enough for the vacuum to form. Each wound has a character, each edge and gully different to that of the next person. Sometimes the vasculature is visible, like threadbare curtains with the light peeping through. Occasionally other layers can be seen, fat and muscle or white bone gleaming in the depths, but no two wounds look the same; each has a story to tell and a little more to teach us.

Sidney had developed painful leaking sores on both legs as a result of poor blood flow, and needed to be monitored by the vascular clinic. He had not been attending recent appointments and had only come this time because his social worker had managed to persuade him.

I was a few months into my first job as a qualified nurse and working on the vascular ward that morning. At midday, Sidney was wheeled in on a hospital trolley from the clinic, accompanied by the vascular nurse specialist clutching his notes.

He transferred himself to the bed and began unwrapping the bandages on his legs, which I could see were already leaking yellow fluid onto the sheet.

'Sidney, why don't you leave them for a while?' the vascular nurse specialist asked. 'We've just removed the maggots and re-dressed them for you.'

'Exactly.' Sidney didn't look up. His fingers picked at the edges of the dressings. 'You've got rid of them.'

'Well they couldn't stay there, Sidney. That's why the ulcers have become infected.'

I hadn't yet received handover and didn't know anything about Sidney. One of the ward's healthcare assistants walked in and asked whether he would like anything for lunch and whether she could take his blood pressure.

'Go away,' he said.

'Let me hand over,' the nurse specialist said, and we moved from the room to a nearby desk where we leant and opened up the notes.

Sidney was still in view; he held strands of bandage between each thumb and forefinger as if he were tying a ribbon into a bow. He shook his head. His hair was grey and he had a beard that was matted at the bottom. Nurses deal with many smells throughout a shift and in the main are pretty immune to them, but the odour from Sidney's infected leg wounds was something different.

The nurse specialist smiled at me and let out a sigh at the same time.

'So, Sidney has been under the vascular team for a while, but unfortunately we haven't seen him in months. Somebody from the community team tried to visit him in sheltered housing, but he wouldn't let them in. He's also in the care of a psychiatric hospital in north London, but I believe he hasn't been engaging with them either.'

I nodded and the nurse continued.

'We were pleased to see him this morning. Sixty-five-year-old gentleman with a history of alcohol misuse, peripheral vascular disease, diabetes and schizophrenia. This morning he attended clinic for a wound dressing. He has bilateral venous leg ulcers that require daily dressings and we have been hoping to scan his legs to look at flow. This morning I had a look at them and could quite clearly see and smell that they are now infected. Unfortunately, certain flies are drawn to warm, smelly leg wounds, since they have a supreme sense of smell. And that's what has happened to poor Sidney. When he came to me, his legs were utterly infested with maggots. Poor chap, it's a vicious cycle: of course no one wants to leave the house to attend the hospital with maggots on their legs.'

'When did this happen?' I asked.

'He's developed the infection over a period of months, but has spent the last few weeks with these tissue-destroying flies laying fifty to three hundred eggs at a time on his skin. Eggs, maggots, pupae, flies; the social worker told me the flat is crawling with flies. It's not a fit place to live. Anyway, we've cleaned the wounds, rid them entirely of the infestation; now we just need to continue to treat the infection. I am hoping he'll allow you to cannulate him and give him intravenous antibiotics and regular wound dressings. If he doesn't, he might lose those legs to gangrene.'

I thanked the nurse specialist for the handover, looked at the drug chart and the doctor's plan and went back in to see Sidney. He was still, very cautiously, trying to unwrap the bandages.

'Hi, Sidney,' I said. 'My name is Molly.'

He held up a finger to silence me.

'I didn't ask you to say anything,' he said. 'When some-one is ready to begin a conversation they will make eye contact with you. Did I make eye contact?'

I waited for him to continue.

He looked up and raised his eyebrows.

'I'm Molly,' I said.

'You've said that.'

He went back to picking at the dressings.

'I've heard you've had quite a time of it.'

He stopped me again, put down the fronds of dressing and made eye contact.

'You've heard wrong. My dad was a fisherman and could tie six thousand different types of knot. Do you know anything about knots?' he said.

'When I was a child, I liked watching magic, so I taught myself how to escape from a few different rope knots.'

'They can be anything you want them to be, can't they?' Sidney said. His fingers were perfectly still and poised in position, holding out two strands of bandage as if he were going to tie me a knot now. 'One minute they're just a bit of rope, the next they are bowlines, the next they might be a blood knot, perfectly controlled between your fingers.'

I nodded.

'Some people think it's just a piece of old rope. They never wait and see what it could become.'

'Why don't you leave those bandages? They'll last a while; the nurse specialist said she had just dressed your legs.' Orangey fluid was seeping through as he finally revealed another layer beneath.

'The nurse specialist took away the maggots. One moment

they're maggots, the next they're flies. I was keeping them. She didn't know anything about it. I have thirteen pupae waiting to hatch on the bedside table at home and I had a whole nest of maggots that now won't fly.'

'I'm sorry, Sidney. We need to make sure those leg wounds are clean and can heal.'

'The maggots were doing that!' he shouted.

In some ways Sidney wasn't wrong. Military surgeons noted the therapeutic effects of maggots on wounds centuries ago, and their subsequent use was successful in treating certain types of wound.

Looking after Sidney became a lesson in timing. Care and conversation had to be meticulously in keeping with his plan for the day.

He told me he had grown up by the sea. His father had been away for long periods of time on his ship, and his mother drank when her husband was away. One evening after school, she had gone to town to do some shopping. Sidney looked in the house for his dad, and then remembered that at this time, before dinner, he was usually to be found working on his boat down by the water. He went to find him, but the boathouse was empty and dark, the boat moored in place, bobbing gently in the shallows. He went further into the boathouse, taking the torch off the hook by the door and shining it against the wood. It was then that he saw his dad's feet.

'He'd hung himself with a noose,' Sidney said as I knelt at his feet, sterile gloves and dressings ready.

'I'm so—' I began. But Sidney held up one finger.

'It wasn't just any type of noose. When I cut him down,

I wasn't able to fathom the knot he had tied. I couldn't undo it with my hands and I didn't want to take the knife to his throat.'

He circled his hand, encouraging me to carry on with the dressing. I began to wash his legs in the papier-mâché bowl of warm water.

'Do you know about knots?' he asked again.

I looked up at him.

'Just a few,' I said.

'Hmm . . .' he replied.

His legs looked a bit better already; he had allowed us to give him intravenous antibiotics, and we were hoping to persuade him to let us apply the vacuum-assisted therapy box today. I wanted to talk to him about that, but didn't interrupt.

'My dad knew how to tie six thousand knots. Just a bit of rope, most people think, but they're not . . .'

Over the next few weeks, Sidney's legs deteriorated. He wouldn't allow us to apply the vacuum-assisted therapy or dress his legs. He needed a long course of regular intravenous antibiotics but wouldn't let us put a more permanent cannula in his arm to deliver them. He wanted to go home; he was worried about the pupae on the bedside table. Social services had deemed his house uninhabitable and it was undergoing fumigation. Soon he didn't want anybody to touch his legs at all, and as a result we were unable to check on them. Psychologists from a local psychiatric unit tried to visit him on the ward, but he wouldn't let them in his room. He was at risk of losing his legs and his life, and so the whole team sat down to discuss his case. Eventually it was decided that in order to give him the best possible chance of keeping both, he would be sectioned under the Mental Health Act. We believed that he lacked the capacity and insight into his condition to make decisions for himself.

I was working at the other end of the ward the day Sidney left, but I saw the porter come to pick him up and wheel him downstairs to the transport waiting to take him to the psychiatric hospital. His bandages were soaked through and a nurse tried to cover them with a blanket. Sidney wouldn't allow it and waved it away. The porter wheeled him slowly, the nurse beside him clutching two big folders full of his medical notes.

As they left the ward, Sidney tilted his head up to his new nurse.

'Do you know anything about knots?' he said.

39

On the television and in the newspapers there was increasing news of people dying at sea and in makeshift camps as they fled war in their homelands. There was no togetherness in watching the news; it seemed as if it would continue whether we watched or not, whether we went to help or didn't. The situation was huge and hopeless and hard to look at.

In February I travelled back to France, but this time to volunteer in the refugee camp in Calais. Even though I had been qualified almost two years, it wasn't until I visited 'the Jungle' that I came to understand fully the final part of the nursing assessment and the importance of exposure.

I left home in the dark one early rain-swept winter morning. Rob helped pack the last of the sleeping bags and shoeboxes in the boot. We kissed goodbye, hugged, and I got in the car. The radio talked of Storm Henry, which was bringing eighty-mile-an-hour gusts across the UK and waves and floods on coastal roads. Dover was seventy miles away. The ferry crossing was an hour and a half. The wipers were on full speed and the roads were empty.

The ferry left on time and I watched as we pulled away

from the dock, street lamps bobbing in the distance, the rain beating hard against the floor-to-ceiling window, the sea white and raging below, waves upturned as if calling for help. A small child screamed and pointed at them. The lighting on board the ship was dim and the floor was heavily carpeted; everything smelt of diesel and air freshener. I rested my head against the shuddering glass and must have fallen asleep, because soon we were docking in France.

Calais was grey and bleak. It felt strange to be arriving in France knowing I wasn't here for a holiday. As I drove away from the ferry, I saw wind turbines spinning maniacally in the gale, stretched out along the coast like emaciated white ghosts. It looked as if nothing else could grow here. A cluster of cranes loomed behind wire fencing, their heads bowed together. In the distance I could see rows of pylons with their steel arms restrained by thick black electrical cabling. I opened the window to let out the stink of diesel and heard the monstrous clank of shipyard pulleys bringing the boats in from the storm.

I closed the window and concentrated on the satnav.

The warehouse was a twenty-minute drive from the ferry terminal. On either side of the long road there was barbed wire with little pieces of torn clothing and blankets stuck on its spikes. I drove through the outskirts of town, past an old lighthouse, a watchtower, a cash-and-carry, and boarded-up seafront restaurants that advertised mussels and clams on ripped, sun-washed posters. I turned off the main road, down a smaller one dotted with warehouses. I had been told to look out for a bright blue building with yellow doors. I found it immediately, a giant sunflower door frame grinning like a clown in the rain.

Inside the warehouse the atmosphere was shining. People in tabards lugged boxes across the floor, smiling, shouting, swigging from steaming mugs of tea, spooning soup into their mouths, and singing along to the radio that was blasting from a speaker decorated with Christmas lights. There were mountains of clothes and shoes and brown boxes labelled with sizes and descriptions, and volunteers were arm-deep within them, pulling items out and inspecting them.

I was welcomed, given tea and put to work on the conveyer-belt-style main table, sifting through trainers to make sure they were good enough to give away, and then sorting them into type and size. We spent hours doing it and the time passed quickly.

As the weather outside worsened, the warmth in the warehouse grew. The heaters glowed red at their filaments. We were warm from sorting, and when we wanted a break, we sat in camping chairs, our feet propped up on pallets, hands cupped around mugs of tea.

In the afternoon I saw a few young women unlocking one of the shipping containers outside. I went to see if they needed any help. The container was stacked floor to ceiling with medical equipment: bandages and stockings, iodine and antiseptic creams. One of the women was reading from a list whilst the other two searched the shelves and collected items in carrier bags. There was a Scottish doctor and two Portuguese nurses. They told me they had been volunteering in the medical caravans in camp, which now needed restocking. I told them I was a nurse and they asked if I wanted to join them in the morning.

We woke early and met in the foyer of the hostel. As I drove us to the camp, I could feel my heart beating very fast in my chest. The CRS, the French riot police, were lined up along the bridge. They were wearing all black, with thick steel-toecap boots and shell-like armour on their backs. They had guns, batons and shields. We drove slowly past them. They looked into the car as we passed but didn't stop us. In the rear-view I saw them start to walk in ordered lines through the muddy field towards the camp. Up ahead I saw a bulldozer on the peripheries arcing its open mouth up towards the slate sky.

As we got closer to the entrance of the camp, we saw that the bulldozer was bringing down a wooden building. Only the bare bones of it were left: its felt skin, the slats and tiles, a large cross that now lay discarded in the mud. It had been the camp church. People stood around watching in silence. The CRS stood on a grassy mound surveying the scene, guns held tightly. There were already spent rubber bullets lying at their feet.

When the bulldozer stopped and the engine was turned off, a woman in flip-flops walked towards the skinless church and picked up the cross. It was heavy; you could see that in the way she bent her legs to heave it onto her shoulders. It was electric blue and wet from the rain. Nobody said anything as she walked back into the camp with it.

We left the car at the entrance and went in. Nobody looked at us; volunteers had been coming and going for months. There were makeshift shops and restaurants lining a muddy path, and people had used wooden pallets to lift their sleeping bags and tarpaulin shelters off the sodden earth. There were oil barrel bonfires everywhere, the black smoke pluming towards the sky, and huddles of men protecting their noses and mouths from it stood around with their hands out, warming them.

We walked deeper into the camp. The medical facility was a lopsided fibreglass caravan half submerged in the mud. It was stocked with hot water, cough sweets and bandages, but most of all, it was warm inside. The air smelt of eucalyptus and clove from the wristbands the other volunteers had been making that morning. The men who visited the caravan had asked for 'mint bands', which were made from cotton bandages dipped in menthol oil, to be used as a decongestant. Wearing these meant that they could stand beside the fires to keep warm without breathing in the toxic black smoke from all the things that shouldn't be burnt on a fire: plastic sheeting and ripped tents. The volunteers who came and went in the medical caravans made hundreds of them; whilst one person tended to a patient, the other would be cutting bandages into strips and leaving them to soak in the oil.

At first I stood and watched the doctor as she assessed a patient. She made sure that they sat far away from the open caravan door and offered them hot water and fruit from a bowl. The men coming through the door all had hunched shoulders, locked tightly in position from shivering all day and all night. They rubbed their hands together; the noise was like dry autumn leaves. They held them between their legs whilst they talked.

Shiz worked as an interpreter in the camp. He could speak five languages and stood in between the two medical caravans helping to translate for us all. Whilst the Scottish doctor tended to the patient, I went outside and brought Shiz a cup of lemon tea. I asked him if he was not freezing standing outside; wouldn't he prefer to come in, sit down and help translate from there? He smiled at me, cupping the hot drink between his gloved hands. He said he couldn't feel the cold any more.

At midday, a young man knocked on the plastic window of the caravan and looked inside nervously. It was raining outside and I could see Shiz laughing with a group of young boys gathered around a black-smoke fire.

'Come in, come in,' the doctor called. She was only young herself but had been qualified a few years and had worked in many different hospitals in the UK. She was confident and listened to everything people told her. 'Hi,' she said. 'I'm Sarah.'

The young man shook her hand.

'I'm Adel.'

'Are you okay?' she asked.

He nodded. It was a big question.

I made him tea.

'There's a storm in England,' Sarah said. 'I think that's why it's so windy today.'

They both looked outside at the grey camp, at the wind

tearing through the shelters. On a piece of corrugated fence somebody had spray-painted the words 'EVERY-BODY WELCOME', with a smiley face beside them. Some of the young men from the Eritrean part of the camp had joined Shiz and the younger boys and they were kicking a half-deflated football around the bonfire, all of them with their hands still in their pockets. Some of the men had wrapped their scarves around their faces to try and stop themselves from inhaling the worst of the smoke.

'How're you feeling?' Sarah asked.

'Very bad,' Adel said. 'It's my chest, I have such a pain in my chest.'

Sarah nodded.

'And my hand as well, I want to show you my hand.'

I hadn't noticed, but now I saw that Adel was keeping one hand tucked beneath his armpit.

'Can I see?' Sarah asked. She put her hands out in front of her, waiting for his.

Slowly he brought his hand down. It was wrapped in dirty bandages, and when the doctor touched it, he bit his front teeth down on his lip.

'It's painful?' she said.

Adel nodded. 'I think it's broken.'

'What happened?' Sarah asked as she began to unwrap the bandage.

'Police . . .' Adel said.

Sarah had been in the camp for two weeks, and most of the injuries she had encountered were from police beatings: streaming eyes from tear gas and fractured eye sockets from baton whacks.

'Where are you from?' she asked.

'Syria,' Adel said. 'From Aleppo.'

'How old are you?' I sat beside him.

'Nineteen.'

'How long did it take you to get here?'

'Three months,' he said. He shook his head and looked down at his feet.

'On foot?' I asked.

'Foot, boat, car. I got to Turkey with my family and carried on without them. I don't know if they are still there, if they are safe. But we had to leave. My dad was shot. If you stay and won't fight, you die.'

Sarah had unwrapped Adel's hand. It was a different colour to the rest of his skin, almost blue-black with bruise.

'Oh Adel,' she said, staring at it. 'You will have to go to hospital. It needs an X-ray, it needs to be set.'

'Can't you fix it?'

Sarah shook her head.

'I'm not going into town,' he said.

The centre of town was dangerous for refugees. Even some of the volunteers helping in the camp had been beaten up. The streets were bare and open; the wind from the sea seemed colder, passing through all that metalwork on the jetty. There was nowhere to hide in the centre of town.

Sarah and Adel looked at each other. There was blood streaked between his fingers and two of his nails were missing.

'What did they do to you?'

Adel shut his eyes.

'They held me down,' was all he said.

'Let me splint the fingers.' Sarah stood up and showed me where everything was whilst she washed the skin on his hand with warm water. She gave him some painkillers and he took an orange from the bowl.

'You'll need help peeling that,' Sarah said.

Adel smiled and shook his head at the orange. I took it from him and peeled it.

Once she had cleaned the skin, splinted the fingers and let me dress Adel's hand, she listened to his chest.

'Are you breathing in that smoke?' she said, and pointed out at the oil-barrel fires.

'It's so cold,' he said. 'I can't remember what it feels like to be warm.'

We gave him a menthol band and Sarah found a scarf in one of the boxes.

'Wear this around your face like the other boys,' she said. 'You have a chest infection. It will only get worse with the smoke and the cold. And come back to us every day if you want to.'

'Thank you,' he said. His good hand held the orange.

Sarah tied the scarf around his neck and I made us all tea. Shiz came in and sat with us. He rubbed his hands together and shivered. They made that same autumn-leaf sound. He and Adel spoke in Arabic. Sarah and I listened and tidied the caravan. The two men laughed, their shoulders relaxed.

On the fourth day, some volunteers asked if we could use my car to drop off supplies to the camp in Dunkirk, over twenty miles away. I agreed, and after breakfast we drove there in silence on a long, straight road, my rear-view mirror blocked by boxes of shoes and sleeping bags.

Dunkirk was worse. When we arrived, the CRS were frisking anybody walking in and out of the camp. We hadn't seen many children in Calais, but here they were everywhere, in oversized wellies and pyjamas. Inside, the camp was drowning in mud. There were discarded sheets of tarpaulin and ripped tents submerged in swamp, splintered duckboards that had once made a path but now lay broken, leading to nowhere. The same black smoke hung in the air; people gathered around upturned oil barrels and threw plastic bottles on the fire to stoke it and try to stay warm. In the distance, I could hear explosions.

We walked slowly through the mud. Some people smiled at us; others didn't. Up ahead there was a clearing; in the middle there was a leafless tree, standing lopsided in the dirt. Strung to every branch was a child's toy: a teddy bear hanging by its neck; a doll, streaked in mud, dangling by its wrist; a monkey with one eye; an owl staring out at the camp, yellow-eyed, tied by its wing to a bare branch.

We delivered some of the boxes and went back to the car to get more. On the way, a little girl leapt from a rain-soaked tent. She hopped on the spot and balanced on one leg to slide her little feet into her wellies. She wobbled and laughed. I held out my hand to steady her; she couldn't have been more than seven years old. She took my hand, and it was the coldest skin I had ever felt. She smiled up at me, slipped into her wellies and then was gone, running, chasing another child further into the camp.

I had tears in my eyes but didn't want to let them fall. We busied ourselves emptying the boot. Two men came and helped us; one of them had his little girl beside him. When all the boxes were out of the car, I noticed that one of my niece's old baby toys was on the back seat. I hadn't remembered it was there. I took it out and knelt beside a gravel-filled puddle with it; the little girl walked over holding her dad's hand by the finger. She had big brown eyes and two little gold studs in her ears. The toy was a plastic tree and a cradle that would swing when you pressed a button. It used to play 'Rock-a-bye Baby' but it had run out of batteries and I didn't have any more.

'Do you know that song?' I asked the man.

He crouched beside us and shook his head. The other man came to watch.

I sang the beginning of the lullaby; he didn't seem to recognize it.

'Will you sing it again?' he said. 'I want to remember it so I can sing it to her back inside the tent.'

I nodded and sang.

Rock-a-bye baby, in the treetop
When the wind blows, the cradle will rock . . .

I tried not to cry. The little girl looked up at me and smiled and smiled, reaching out for the toy. I tried not to think of the tree I'd seen inside the camp.

When the bough breaks, the cradle will fall
And down will come baby, cradle and all.

40

The next time I was in France, it was a different world. Paris was a beautiful glossy mess, an oil painting half drowned beneath the Seine, which had risen to its highest level in thirty years. Rob and I were on a weekend away.

One evening the sky was catacomb black. Notre-Dame cathedral was illuminated by hundreds of tiny fires blazing fiercely through its latticed facade. Rob took my hand as we walked beside the Seine towards Pont Neuf. A bronze statue shone with rain above us. We stood on the bridge overlooking the river; it is the oldest bridge in Paris, the heart of the city.

'Mol,' Rob said.

I turned around.

He was on one knee on the rain-wet bridge, a hand outstretched, asking me to marry him. I said yes.

Back home, Dad was almost healed from his heart operation. He was walking the dog and swimming twice a week at the pool we used to go to every weekend. The swimming pool was up a hill, and as he walked, he no longer felt out of breath, his heart valve fixed; instead, though, he felt pain in his leg that made him stop and sit on the grit bins to let it pass. The pain continued, and almost a year later Dad's foot had gone cold.

That morning, we drove to A&E. Dad could hardly walk with the pain travelling up his leg; it had kept him awake all night. We stopped and waited outside the department as he caught his breath. The day was barely light yet; a low winter fog covered the trees and the cars in the car park. Slowly we walked through the swing doors.

The triage nurse took Dad's observations. His blood pressure was far too high. They did blood tests and one of the results came back positive, revealing that a blood clot might have formed at some point and been broken down in his body.

Dad rubbed at his calf, massaging the soft muscle to try and make the pain go away. It eased as we sat waiting. The nurse told him they could admit him to a bed but that he wouldn't be able to have a scan until the next morning. Dad wanted to go home and rest, so we drove back with an appointment for a scan of his leg booked for early the next day.

The next day I was on shift at the hospital. At ten in the morning, the phone rang on the unit; it was the nurse from Dad's local hospital. His scan had revealed aneurysms and blood clots running down both legs, and he was being rushed to my hospital. I thanked her and said I would meet him in A&E downstairs. I spoke to Mum. Neither of us knew quite what it meant. Mum said she would leave work now and come straight to the hospital.

In a side room, the vascular doctor examined Dad's leg. The skin was cold and dusky blue in colour. He lifted the leg up and the blood quickly drained, leaving it white and translucent.

'Positive,' the doctor said to the air. His colleague made a note.

'Positive for what?' I asked.

'Buerger's . . .' He turned away from me and talked to the other doctor. They spoke in quiet tones. I looked at Dad, one hand laid across his forehead, the other resting beneath his head on the hospital trolley.

'What is it, Doctor?' I said.

'Critical limb ischaemia,' he replied, already looking past me through the door to the busy emergency department beyond. 'The leg might be salvageable. I'm getting in touch with my consultant.' He nodded to Dad and he and his colleague left.

'Jesus . . .' Dad said, staring up at the ceiling.

'What is it?' I went to him and took his hand.

'The foot's gone dead, hasn't it? They're gonna have it off.'

'We don't know anything yet, Dad. Let's wait and see what the consultant says.'

'Well, Mum's always telling me I need to lose weight . . .'

'Dad!' I said. We both laughed, but I couldn't tell by the end if we were laughing or crying.

Dad was admitted to the vascular ward I had worked on as a newly qualified nurse, the ward in which I had met Sidney with his leg wounds. Mum arrived and we told her the news and that we were waiting for more information. There was a clock on the wall with a bare white face. Time didn't move as we waited for the doctors to return.

I put my hands on Dad's cold foot. He said it was no longer sore but it felt heavy. It was pale and grey at the toes. I tried to feel for a pulse on the top of his foot, around the ankle, where an artery lay. There was nothing; the foot was cold and pulseless.

We stared at the clock.

Mum rang my sister.

Finally two consultants arrived. They stood in the doorway and introduced themselves, and despite their smiles, the room felt cloaked in shadow.

'We need to get a scan,' one of them said. He wore a suit and leant both his arms on the bed. He looked at Dad before examining his foot. 'A scan of the pipework in your legs will show us just how bad they are.'

'They're bad?' Mum asked.

The other doctor nodded. He held his hands clasped gently in front of him, his tie tucked into his shirt.

'Mr Case, from your scan at the other hospital, it does appear you have significant blockages running up and down both legs.'

Dad nodded.

'The leg is now in danger.'

'Critical limb ischaemia.' I repeated the words I had heard. The foot was dead, and if left any longer without circulation, it might have to be amputated.

'Yes.' The doctor looked at us all. 'We'll get you scanned and get an angiogram to look inside the vessels. Then we will know what we are dealing with and how to proceed.'

'Today?' Mum said.

'All as soon as possible. We might not have a lot of time.' He laid his hands on Dad's foot and lower leg as if calming the surface of the water.

'I can't lose my leg, Doc,' Dad said quietly. 'I have to walk my daughter down the aisle this year.'

'Dad . . .' I tried to stop him, but the words were out and I had to leave the room, the tears coming uncontrollably. Mum came out with me and Dad was left with the two doctors telling him they would do their very best to save his leg.

Outside, I cried on Mum's shoulder and she held me close. I shut my eyes and thought of the fern Dad had plucked from the wet woods when I was a child, the one that we had carefully carried home and replanted in the garden to watch it grow.

The angiogram revealed that Dad's legs were riddled with blockages and there were very few remaining vessels they could use to try and bypass the obstructions. They would, of course, try. In the gloom of the vascular ward, they talked him through the risks of having the surgery: catastrophic bleeding, amputation, death. Dad signed the form. He would be taken to surgery the next day to try and save his leg.

Before he was wheeled down to theatre, one of the consultants came to see him again. Dad was in his hospital gown, he had a cannula in his arm with intravenous fluids since he was being starved prior to surgery, and he had taken his dentures out in preparation.

'Doctor,' he said, shaking the consultant's hand over the bars of his hospital bed. 'I want to know . . . Did the scan show you something you could use; is there anything there?'

He wanted some hope, some knowledge of what he would wake up to on the other side. I could barely listen to the answer.

The doctor held his gaze.

'We're hopeful,' he said, and squeezed Dad's out-stretched hand. 'We'll see you in theatre, Mr Case.' He smiled and left.

Dad rested his head heavily back on the pillow and closed his eyes. It was all he needed to hear before being taken away.

Dad's femoral bypass operation took a long time. He went down to theatre in the afternoon and didn't come out until late at night. We all went home and waited. The night was freezing cold; it was the middle of January and there was frost on the garden gate lit up by the blueness of the moon.

Just before eleven, the phone rang and I ran outside to get mobile reception. The pavement was searing cold. A muscle memory from my childhood came careering back to me through the soles of my feet. I was a child once more, having my swimming pool verrucas burnt off by a nurse in the GP's surgery wielding a canister of frozen nitrogen. For years afterwards I felt the cigarette-burn holes in the soles of my feet like a stigmata, but as I grew older, the memory faded until I had forgotten them entirely. Standing on the pavement that night, awaiting news of Dad, I felt the coldness once more.

'It was a long, complex operation,' the surgeon said.

I pressed the phone hard against my ear.

'His vessels were like glass; we had to be very careful . . .'

I imagined the room full of blue-scrubbed people; a theatre I knew so well. Sterile drapes, clamps, suction, the smell of singed skin cut open to reveal the pipework within.

'We are happy with how it went,' he continued. 'He's in recovery now. The foot is warm, there are pulses; we're satisfied we have re-routed his circulation.'

I rested against the cold garden wall, lifted my bare soles from the pavement.

'Thank you,' I said. 'Thank you.' It was all I could say.

At home, Dad's leg healed badly. The wound seams split and became infected from his groin to his ankle. For the next four months I went round two or three times a week to clean and dress the wound. I taught Mum how to do it when I wasn't there, and spoke to the tissue viability nurses at work for advice. At first they told me to use honey on the wound, then iodine, and when it still wouldn't heal, they told me that since the circulation in Dad's legs was so poor, it would most likely never heal at all.

I didn't tell Dad this. When I went round to clean the wound, we read each other poetry. Dad wanted me to read his favourite poem to him aloud, and with his leg propped on a pillow, the sterile water and gauze laid out ready, he listened and looked out at the oak trees in the garden with the wood pigeons swaying between the leaves.

The wound was deep and the edges far apart. As the weeks went on, we tried different ways of getting it to heal. Some weeks we re-dressed it frequently, not allowing it to become wet; other times we left it longer, letting the iodine or honey soak into the skin. The good skin around the wound became stark white and wrinkled, as if I was doing more harm than good.

Then one day, kneeling over the wound with the bedside light angled to see it more closely, I realized the sides were beginning to close. The skin was pinker than it had been before and had already started to join together on one side.

'Dad,' I said, looking up at him. 'I think it's healing.'

We were all patient, and continued as we had done for so many months. Every time I took off the dressing, I felt my heart beating faster, fearful that what I had seen was not really there, or that it would have deteriorated again and reopened or become infected while I'd been away.

Each time, Dad asked me how it looked, and I told him to be quiet, to let me clean it and inspect it under the light so I could see fully before saying anything. Each week it looked better. The deep hole it had once been was shallower now, and I could see the good wound bed beneath rising upwards, a sturdy vascular foundation in which a scab and then a scar could finally form.

41

By the spring, Dad's leg had healed and all that was left was a long, twisting scar that curled down his inner leg like a space observatory photo of a river cutting across the earth. It looked like the Colorado River we had flown over, bucking and jolting through the turbulence of the Grand Canyon, that long-ago summer holiday. In the sun-glint the surface of the river became a mirror, an optical illusion offering up a reflection of the sun and the upper sky that lay above.

Dad's healed skin was left smoother than it had been, hairless and soft to the touch, like new skin. He walked with a stick, was slow, but he was back on his feet again and able to go out.

In May, our wedding came. It was flower-filled on a blustery spring day. My veil was long and the wind swept it high into the air like a feather. We were married outside, beneath a white sun, in twelve acres of English garden. My sister's little girls, aged four and two, held white gypsophila tied with ribbon, and afterwards ran and played, exploring the woodland, the greenhouse, the herb garden and the Tudor knot garden, where everything was aligned in perfect symmetry.

I walked towards Rob, veil streaming; I could smell the

sweetness from my bouquet: pink veronicas, peach-coloured roses, eucalyptus leaves and ferns gathered around the edges. Beside me, Dad walked with his stick. I held on to him and he held on to me. Our footsteps were perfectly together, slow, heel and ball on the earth at the same time so that we wouldn't leave it, and if we did, it would be together.

In the warm glow of the garden tent, we raised our glasses. The room was hung with photographs from mine and Rob's travels, all held together with string.

Dad stood and spoke. He talked about my childhood, the woodland walks in the rain, swimming, jazz music. And then he read the Stephen Spender poem 'To My Daughter'.

> Bright clasp of her whole hand around my finger,
> My daughter, as we walk together now,
> All my life I'll feel a ring invisibly
> Circle this bone with shining: when she is grown
> Far from today as her eyes are far already.

> When I was a boy and I would see scary things in the
> news, my mother would say to me, 'Look for the
> helpers. You will always find people who are helping.'
>
> Fred Rogers

A month later, it was a warm summer evening in June. South of the river, people were sitting outside pubs, having a drink and eating from stalls, sheltered beneath the ironwork roof of Borough Market. The river was calm, Southwark Cathedral glowed from the inside, the roads were busy with black cabs and buses.

Just after ten p.m., a van drove across the bridge. It picked up speed and mounted the pavement, swerving into pedestrians and running them down. The van continued on towards Borough Market. Three young men got out of the vehicle and ran towards the pubs and the market area. They were armed with twelve-inch ceramic knives with pink blades and pink handles, tied to their wrists with leather straps. They shouted as they ran.

At seven minutes past ten, ambulances were dispatched, police just a minute later. On the streets, people ran in every direction, crying, screaming, throwing crates and chairs at the men wielding the knives. The attackers slashed frantically at anybody they could see; the subsequent knife wounds on the victims' bodies were random: face, neck, chest, legs, arms.

By sixteen minutes past ten, all three attackers had been shot dead by armed police.

London hospitals worked tirelessly through the night, off-duty staff coming in to help in emergency departments, operating theatres and the wards where patients were admitted.

I worked on the HDU in the aftermath.

Two days later, I arrived at seven in the morning. A police guard sat on a chair outside the unit; he was tall and thin, with freckles across his nose. He held his hat in his hands and leant his head against the wall. It looked as if he hadn't slept in days.

'How are you?' I asked.

He smiled, as if the question was too big.

'Tired.' He sighed and wiped his eyes. 'It's all right, I'm supposed to be relieved in a bit.'

'Bed soon,' I said.

He nodded and rested his head once more.

I pushed the door to make my way into the staff room.

The day staff were sipping coffee and watching the news: reporters talking outside the hospital entrances around the city that we knew so well. Some of the night staff came in and sat down, resting their heads on their colleagues' shoulders, bird's-nest hair and creased uniforms.

Eight people had been killed and almost fifty were injured.

Out on the unit, we looked after people with chest

wounds, collapsed lungs requiring chest drains, rib fractures, and blood accumulating in their chests from punctured lungs. These patients slept, and when they woke needed morphine to cope with the pain. Many of them still had blood crusted in their hair and beneath their fingernails despite having been helped to wash by the nurses.

One shift left and the next continued, and when eight o'clock in the evening came, the same would happen again, and again the next morning, eight o'clock, coffee and toast, eight in the evening, coffee and toast, a baton passed between outstretched hands, tracing the arc and loop of the figure of it, eight in the morning, eight in the evening, on the roadside with the sun going down, in the ambulances, in the resus department, the CT scanner, the operating theatre, on the ward with the sun breaking through the night clouds.

Acknowledgements

Thank you to my family for allowing me to write about our lives. I owe everything I've learnt and pursued so far to the knowledge you've imparted along the way and the experiences that you've given me.

Thank you to my mum for her wisdom and her time spent reading early versions, helping me to edit; thank you to my sister for her insight and expert mother and baby knowledge; to my dad who I know feels bemused that a whole book could be written about him, of course it could, he is the most fascinating person we know; and to Rob whose patience, love and understanding of both me and the story I wanted to tell, has helped me finish this book.

Thank you: Zoë Waldie who inspired me from the moment I met her and has guided me ever since, Mary Mount who transformed the book into what it always should have been, to Dr Steele, Dr Glizevskaja, and Dr Dhillon who enlightened me with their cardiac knowledge, to the surgeons that operated on my dad, my nursing colleagues who I have learnt so much from, many of them nursing Dad back to health, and who in those days at the hospital let me simply be a daughter. And thank you to the patients, for giving me this incredible career and letting me be part of their own stories.